Train Your Brain

Bettina M. Jasper

Train Your Brain

Mental and Physical Fitness

Meyer & Meyer Sport

Original title: Brainfitness : Denken und Bewegen
© 1998 by Meyer & Meyer Verlag, Aachen/Germany
Translated by Paul Chilvers-Grierson

Die Deutsche Bibliothek – CIP Einheitsaufnahme

Jasper, Bettina M.:
Train your brain : mental and physical fitness / Bettina M. Jasper.
[Transl.: Paul Chilvers Grierson].
– Aachen : Meyer und Meyer, 1999
Dt. Ausg. u.d.T.: Jasper, Bettina M.: Brainfitness
ISBN 3-89124-531-9

© 1999 by Meyer & Meyer Sport, Aachen
Olten (CH), Vienna, Oxford,
Québec, Lansing/ Michigan, Adelaide, Auckland, Johannesburg
e-mail: verlag@meyer-meyer-sports.com
http://www.meyer-meyer-sports.com
Cover design: Walter J. Neumann, N&N Design-Studio, Aachen
Cover photo: Michael von Fisenne, Fotoagentur, Aachen
Figures: see sublines in the text
Type exposure and cover exposure: frw, Reiner Wahlen, Aachen
Printed and bound in Germany by
Burg Verlag & Druck, Gastinger GmbH und Co. KG, Stolberg
ISBN 3-89124-531-9
Printed in Germany

Contents

Foreword

This book is designed primarily for Physical Education trainers and sports teachers working with adult groups. Those working with children or young people in schools or clubs can also integrate many of the exercises and games into their own teaching programmes, but should in some cases choose modified versions. Brain trainers who run courses or work with unchanging groups will find ideas to enrich mental training by including exercises or combined thinking and exercise tasks in their lessons.

The examples have been consciously combined with a number of suggestions for variations. This is to encourage creativity and willingness to change on the one hand. On the other hand it enables adaptation of the exercises to groups of differing abilities and ages.

Variations in the use of equipment, adding or leaving out obstacles, changing the pace, narrowing or widening the space for moving around in etc. offer more flexibility in altering the degree of difficulty of individual tasks and exercises.

Providing a range of variations also makes it possible to adapt to varying locations. Similar exercises can be carried out in halls or outside where there is plenty of space, or in an altered form in more cramped conditions such as in meeting or seminar rooms.

The examples shown here are based on years of experience in gymnastics and sport on the one hand and brain performance training on the other. The author's involvement in both led her to increasingly combine them.

At this point I would like to thank the "Deutscher Turner-Bund"(German Gymnastics Association), which in the last few years gave me the opportunity to make more and more intensive use of events and training courses to present brain training, to arouse interest in it and to test and develop new combinations of thinking and exercise.

As a result, today this subject is an integral part of the work of sports clubs and associations to the extent that there are now a significant number of people qualified in both fields.

My thanks go also to the Klausenbach Memory Clinic in Nordrach (Black Forest) and its training team for their cooperation and technical support as well as their permission to reproduce the "Nousknacker" playing cards developed there in a scientific environment.

I also thank the "Museum of the Cultural History of the Hand" in Wolnzach, Bavaria for permission to use an illustration of the "hand man".

Bettina M. Jasper

1 Brain Fitness: Mental and Physical Fitness – a Topic for Sport

In our performance oriented society, mental fitness is a topic for all age groups. The demands in education and career life are enormous. We have to remain flexible, train ourselves further, perhaps retrain several times in our lifetime and never stop learning. A quick grasp of new things is just as necessary as constant adaptation to new situations.

Apart from that, people get older and want to retain a high quality of life for as long as possible. For this a certain degree of competence and independence is indispensable. Nobody wants lapses in their ability to think and remember things, for everyone wants to be able to make their own decisions about matters affecting themselves.

Nevertheless, the number of - especially older - people with brain function disorders in connection with various illnesses is growing. The fear of Alzheimer disease and similar illnesses is also increasing. The media and advertising add to this. A number of publications deal with the brain and many pharmaceutical companies advertise products to improve blood circulation in the brain and increase thinking, memory and concentration ability.

General health consciousness is extending more and more to the brain and involving mental as well as physical aspects.

An efficient supply of blood to the brain is indispensable for mental fitness. Blood circulation can be influenced not only through medication but especially through exercise. Mental performance increases when thinking is accompanied by movement. Even going for a walk increases the rate of circulation by c. 14 %.

Exercise and thinking are so closely linked, as science has proven, that sports experts are now embracing the topic more than ever before. New training and advanced training courses are being developed in this field. Cooperation between entities in sport on the one hand and medicine and information psychology on the other is becoming more common. It is clear that now already much good is being done for the brain in the training sessions of clubs and other sports organisations, but we are not always aware of this.

For that reason this book contains not only theoretical background, such as the structure and function of the brain, but also numerous examples of exercises which can be included in training sessions and used there to consciously train the brain. Some of these are well known games and exercises, a number of which have been slightly changed and varied to provide effective training of the brain. Active breaks that lead to better circulation in the brain as well as increased awakeness and ability to absorb information and that are also fun can be included not only in training sessions but also in daily club life, at meetings and social gatherings or on trips and excursions. If at the same time attentiveness and creativity are increased and many new ideas developed, the aim has been more than fulfilled.

Mental fitness will continue to be of increasing significance in sport for all age groups.

2 Brain Training – Why and for Whom?

2.1 The Flood of Information

Every day in today's industrial society people have to take in and process – voluntarily or involuntarily – huge amounts of information. Usually, it starts when they wake up. The radio alarm drones news and music. An uninterrupted flow of further information follows: Newspapers, television programmes, private meetings about commitments and plans for the coming day, requirements, instructions, drafts etc. at work.

In our free time too, especially in clubs and organisations, nothing works without an exchange of information. Talking to each other, training sessions, meetings, organising events, contributions to club publications, planning the training programmes, preparing one's own training sessions, additional training about the latest scientific evidence in the field of gymnastics and sport ... The same applies to other organised sport and leisure activities or the regular organisation of courses for training brain performance.

Some information is only briefly processed and exchanged and can then be forgotten once the event has passed, e.g. an agreement about a replacement for next week's session. Once the session has been carried out as agreed, the information can be removed from one's memory. Other things should be retained for as long as possible and be recallable, e.g. information one reads that according to the latest sports health studies a certain exercise should be carried out differently to the way it was done many years ago when one was in training oneself.

Human knowledge is increasing at a phenomenal rate. In the 16th century it was still possible for a single person to learn the total knowledge available to man.

Today nobody could or would want to claim to really know everything. An additional problem is that things we learn today can be completely out of date tomorrow or the next day.

In sport in particular there are numerous examples that physical education teacher training done years ago, a sports degree or another qualification is no guarantee for all time that high quality and correct physical training can be provided. "Circling the head" or the "pocket knife" are just two examples of exercises that used to be considered good and correctly taught and were included in the repertoire of many "old hands" amongst the PE trainers. They all had to learn again and have found that according to more recent studies these two are exercises that damage people's health. The list could be extended continually. The fact that after only a few years, half of what we have learnt in a certain field is out of date, is referred to as the "halflife". In medicine this halflife is currently about four and a half years.

Many of those involved in gymnastics and sport on an honorary basis, whether practically or in organisation and administration, have been so for more than four and a half years. That means they must continually absorb and process new information in order to meet current demands. This is expected of them in addition to the many demands placed on them by their careers and their private spheres. And for professional sportsmen and sportswomen who are involved with movement in clubs or studios it is an absolute necessity to be up to date.

In order to handle all this, what a person needs most is his or her brain. All thinking and planning takes place in this human control centre. Now, there are some people who seem to have no difficulty at all in dealing with many different kinds of burdens and solving problems at work as easily as they fullfil the expectations of their family.

Usually, these are the same people who not only take on honorary positions in clubs but actively carry out these roles. Such people work more productively than others. Their day seems to have at least 48 hours, and in spite of the great amount of activity with a high success rate, to the amazement of others they are well balanced and satisfied. There are such people. Nevertheless, not everyone can claim to cope with everything so easily.

One of the secrets is that some people can deal with information more quickly and can therefore think, plan and decide more quickly than others. Mentally fit people can be up to four times faster than mentally inert colleagues.

Such mental fitness can be trained - just like physical fitness. Only being able to think slowly is no more a matter of fate than having a low level of physical stamina.

2.2 Mental Training in Everyday Llife

Training of the brain does not always take place consciously and in a deliberate manner. Daily life generally provides a high degree of signals and thus impulses for the brain. Anyone who is physically and mentally active, interested in many different things and has much contact with others is in a good position to be and remain mentally on top of things.

Many believe that their job already provides sufficient training for mental agility. That may be true for some fields, but in general the demands we make of ourselves at work are relatively one sided and deliberate.

Even when there are a number of varying activities in our day, we usually have a certain rhythm. Problems and aspects of our work recur at certain periods just as do people with whom we work.

Organised leisure activity, especially in clubs, often provides a healthy balance. Active membership in a club is not a guarantee, but it is certainly a positive factor for mental fitness. Anyone who is active in a gymnastics or sports club is generally active on a regular basis and not just occasionally.

The positive effects of exercise on the functionality of the brain will be covered in more detail later in the book.

Being in a club also forces one to deal with situations and information, to make decisions, to fit in with people and situations. The group, contact with other people, is unavoidable in club life. Conversation – and linked with this the processing of information – is always an aspect of coming together in a group.

And yet club members and other people organised in groups have problems with the performance of their brains in daily life. Have you also found yourself in such situations?

- You want to call an acquaintance who lives nearby to ask them to take you with them in their car tomorrow to the meeting point for a hike. The person has only been in your group a few weeks and you do not know their phone number. So you look it up in the phone book and call. It is engaged. As you go to dial again a few minutes later, you cannot remember the number and have to look it up again.

- You are driving on the motorway in an unfamiliar area to attend a seminar for PE teachers. You know the name of the town, but it is not on any of the many signs you see. Before you have properly registered all the signs and decided which route to take at the motorway junction, you have passed it.

- You have finally got around to carrying out a task that you have been planning a long time and which requires the use of your grey matter – writing an article for the club newsletter, reading an article on sport in a specialist magazine, putting together the annual plan for your department ... When you finally sit down to make a start, your concentration is gone and your mind is blank.

- At the AGM of your club a committee candidate is introduced to you whom you have never seen before. You talk to them for several minutes. As you say goodbye for the meantime and turn to talk with others, you can no longer remember their name.

- Your group plans to present a dance at a large event. First the concept is presented, the movements and choreography seem to be very effective. But now it comes down to practising the details. Again and again you catch yourself moving in the wrong direction, or you have the movement after next in your mind. Each time you manage to save the situation at the last minute, but gradually others in the group start to complain. Typical, always the same people who have to go their own way! And you have made such an effort, but it just won't stay in your mind.

These are just a few typical daily situations that happen to everyone, even when they lead active lives, don't you agree? Increasing use of technology and changing habits mean that many training possibilities of earlier years are becoming increasingly rare in daily life. Who multiplies in their head when there are pocket calculators available? Why should I remember appointments when I have an electronic organiser which is simple and more reliable? Why set up a board game on the table and look for someone to play with when I can quickly click a computer game and don't have to persuade someone else to play with me?

Depending on the type and amount of mental activity in one's daily life, it is recommendable for all age-groups to do deliberate brain training additionally in order to make the most use of our brain capacity, for often great potential lies unused here. Whether you are a woman manager or a houseman, a pensioner or a student - brain training makes sense for everyone and contributes to better and easier handling of everyday situations.

Conscious brain training, however, is not the only influencing factor in regard to mental fitness. Also important is the influence of other factors such as nutrition, exercise, sleep, as well as the social situation. Healthy nutrition, sufficient exercise, restful sleep and being with other people are also part of a training programme for mental fitness.

The functionability of the brain has been proven to have a major influence on one's ability to cope with life's situations, on the quality of life and on life expectancy. It is definitely worth not just concentrating one's health consciousness purely on physical aspects, but at the same time keeping an eye on the brain.

2.3 Mental Fitness and Age

The days when people believed mental fitness declined with increasing age are over. Today it is known that age alone does not determine the level of mental flexibility, but rather a whole combination of factors. These include biological, psychological, social and mental influences.

Figure 1 shows how mental fitness changes with increasing age. Here mental fitness particularly means intelligence, memory, concentration and endurance. The diagram shows average values for individual changes in the various phases of life. According to this illustration, the individual mental peak is reached at about 12 to 16 years (independent of absolute comparative values!).

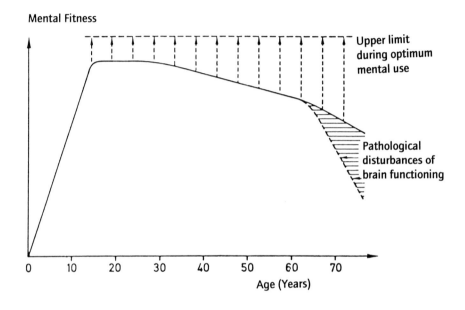

Figure 1: Mental fitness in relationship to age - average changes (from Lehrl, Siegfried / Fischer, Bernd / Lehrl, Maria; Series Gehirntraining: Gejo-Leitfaden. Ein Überblick über Gehirn-Jogging - Grundlagen und Anwendungen, Vless Verlag, Ebersberg, 1990, page 31)

Insufficient and excessive demand on mental activity are considered the main reasons for the decline in mental fitness after age 25/30.

The next bend in the mental fitness curve after 60 is explained by a lack of stimulation (after ending an active career) on the one hand and an increase in disorders of the heart and circulatory system of this age group on the other hand. In addition, at this age disturbances in brain metabolism and circulation often reduce mental fitness further.

In the coming years this situation is expected to change. Increased mobility, changes in our jobs, the necessity to retrain at an advanced age, increased long term unemployment and new patterns of the working life are just some of the factors that will come to bear here.

Health conscious living and prevention rather than cure in all phases of life cannot eradicate illness, but deliberate training and mental and physical activity can reduce the risk factors and the probability of a loss of mental fitness at an advanced age.

The brain ages above all in those places which receive no training. At Helsinki University it has been proven that under natural conditions of aging, the functionability of the brain is the most important influence on life expectancy. Thus a higher level of mental fitness is often coupled with higher life expectancy while amongst those with lower mental fitness the death rate is much higher than in the average population.

Increased education about the connection between life expectancy, quality of life and brain performance in the media on the one hand and the rapid increase in dementing illnesses on the other are certainly reasons why more and more people are turning their attention to their brains and observing themselves more closely, but also developing an increasing fear of loss of ability when they are older. Increasing numbers of people of all ages are also taking the next step and taking up deliberate training of their brains.

We humans are not damned to wait passively until the development shown in Figure 1 finally takes place. The dotted line clearly shows that it is worth staying active. For a person who trains during a lifetime can, if the mind is used optimally, maintain their personal brain fitness at the upper limit, which they once attained at the age of 12 to 16. Even if in certain life phases drops in mental fitness have been registered, it is still worth it - regardless at what age - to begin with new training. Retention and/or improvement in brain performance can take place at any time.

3 Brain Training and Exercise

3.1 Effects of Physical Training on Mental Performance

For a long time now the term sport has no longer been equated only with internationally regulated competitive systems which have as their objective victories and records and are based on a high level of physical fitness. Leisure time and group sport, fitness consciousness, health oriented physical training and above all psychomotorics have led to exercise being understood as something comprehensive in all these fields. A combination of physical, mental, social and emotional components can be assumed. The principle of unity of body and mind is establishing itself more and more and being used more and more.

The relationship between body and mind may be a platitude, nevertheless the results of scientific research are amazing. Exercise increases mental fitness! Research clearly shows that when physical and mental activity occur simultaneously, mental fitness is higher than during physical inactivity. Experiments in which test persons sat on a cycle ergometer and concurrently worked at a computer showed that they solved the tasks on the screen much more successfully than when the same persons worked on these tasks without accompanying physical training. During exercise the short term memory capacity increased to 20 % more than at rest.

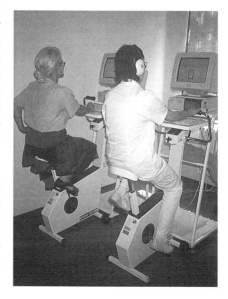

Sporting activity in the sense of the above mentioned comprehensive understanding is generally considered a stimulatory factor which supports perceptive and motional behaviour during the day and thus also - in this connection - planning and thinking.

There is, however, a further link between exercise and thinking. The activation level of a person as a deciding factor of mental fitness can be influenced in various ways, including through exercise. Exercise is considered an activation optimiser. As a rule it can be assumed that the activation level rises during exercise and falls during rest. For this reason, it is easier to think in motion than at physical rest.

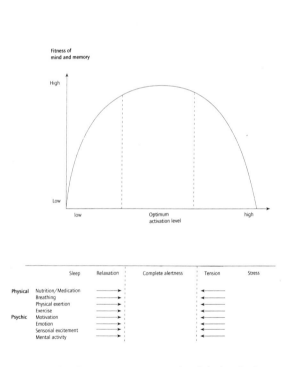

Figure 2.
(from: Lehrgang "Geistige Fitness" by Prof. Dr. med. Bernd Fischer / Dr. med. Bernhard Dickreiter, Hirt Institut, Winterthurerstr. 338, CH-8062 Zürich, Tel.: 0041-1-321 10 20, Fax: 0041-1-321 34 18 cf.: Lehrl, Siegfried / Fischer, Bernd / Lehrl, Maria; Series Gehirntraining: Gejo-Leitfaden. Ein Überblick über Gehirn-Jogging - Grundlagen und Anwendungen, Vless Verlag, Ebersberg, 1990, page 41).

Relationship between activation level (= level of nervous excitement) and fitness of mind and memory. Below these are the physical and psychic levels through which the activation level can be moved.

This illustration shows how the activation level (general state of nervous excitement) influences mental fitness. Fitness is greatest when one is fully alert. On a higher level of general nervous excitement, on the other hand, it is reduced again. That corresponds to people's subjective perception. Under high tension the ability to solve problems suffers, equally brain performance is not at its best in a completely relaxed state.

Alertness is the magic word for those who want to move from a relaxed starting situation to high mental fitness. In this respect, exercises to train one's sense of balance are very useful because they encourage alertness and thus increase the activation level. On the other hand, it is useful to practise relaxing techniques when one is tense or under stress in order to reach an optimum state for mental performance.

A physically well trained person needs much less of his maximum strength to carry out everyday tasks such as carrying shopping or climbing stairs than a person in worse physical shape. Anyone who has to use a great deal of physical strength all day long in order to carry out everyday tasks is more likely to be tired in leisure time and less keen on mental exertion than a trained person who copes with daily life effortlessly.

Animal research has shown that exercise leads to a higher degree of synapses (link between two nerve cells) than does physical rest. With more synapses a person can react more quickly and thus become more mentally flexible.

General endurance training that is matched to age and fitness levels always has a positive effect on brain performance. For this reason all endurance sports such as running, hiking, walking, cycling, swimming, skiing etc. are useful for mental fitness. Excessive physical training, however, should be avoided as it leads to a reduction in thinking performance.

A physical strain of 25 Watts (as for example during a normal walk) leads to improved blood circulation in the brain of c. 14%. At 100 Watts, i.e. four times the strain, it only improves by a further 11 %. According to American research 25 Watts is a good measure in order to reach optimum performance during or shortly after this physical exercise.

This means that even a little exercise considerably increases blood circulation in the brain. Even the conscious imagining of exercise that is not put into practice at all increases blood circulation in the brain. Intensely thinking "I am now raising my right arm" causes a measurable increase in blood supply to the brain without the movement actually taking place. This discovery can be used especially with people whose movements are restricted!

Blood circulation in the brain can be deliberately promoted through certain exercises. The representation of the body surface in the surface of the cerebum shows this clearly.

The motoric Homunculus (lat. the little man reflecting movement) shows through comparative size how well particular parts of the body surface are represented in the brain surface (the somatomotoric cortex).

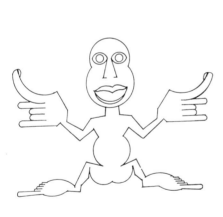 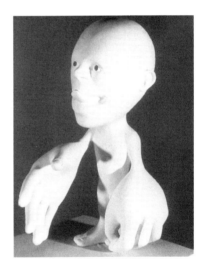

Figure 3. Motoric Homunulus (cf. Mod. nach Schomburg, E.-D. / Kuhnt, U.; Hirnfunktion transparent. Funktionelle Anatomie des Gehirns. Information zum Thema Gehirn 4, Cassella Riedel, u. Fischer B. / Mosmann, H.; Praxishandbuch für Gehirntrainer, Nordrach 1994)

Photo right: "Hand man", with kind permission of the Museum of the Cultural History of the Hand, Wolnzach, Bavaria.

Thus fine motoric exercises, in particular involving fingers and hands, have an especially positive effect on thinking capacity. But also movement of the mouth – e.g. when speaking, singing or chewing ... – improves circulation. Movement of the eye muscle is also effective in this way.

Exercise also makes people feel more relaxed and balanced and thus increases their feeling of well being. This feeling of well being is in turn a prerequisite for a high level of mental fitness.

3.2 Exercise and Thinking in Combination

In almost all forms of physical movement perception is also involved, albeit to varying degrees and in varying fields. Often coordinative abilities are also required, such as reaction, balance, orientation, rhythm, adaptation. In this way the brain and thinking are trained in many ways. Thus combined, i.e. in the linking of exercise and thinking, exercises are correspondingly more effective.

If for example you tap on the table with your fingers, the improving effect of this movement on your circulation is unarguable. When you tap your fingers, you can more or less switch off your thinking and the effect is realised through the movement alone. The effectiveness of such an exercise can be increased if the task "tapping the fingers" is supplemented with another task which requires accompanying thinking – for example tapping them in a certain order or counting how many times you are tapping them.

Such exercises requiring simultaneous processing of information are very popular in gymnastics. Transforming exercises into one's own physical activity requires mental performance. That becomes clear for example when in gymnastics exercises coordinative abilities are required, such as when dance steps including the complete choreography have to be learnt or when in group games the rules have to be understood and then followed. Fast reactions train the brain just as much as adjusting to a situation, learning to use equipment or fitting in with a partner or team.

Sportive movement, especially gymnastics, is as a rule also a form of brain training. Sometimes it requires only a slight change in the exercise or in the

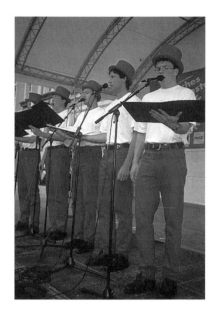

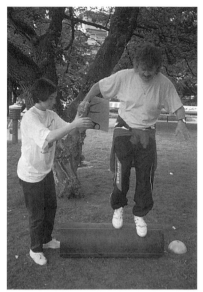

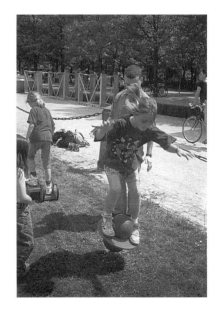

sequence of the lesson to turn a "mere" physical training session into brain training. In many cases the cognitive level (fast absorption and processing of information) and the coordinative level (fast and situational transformation of planned action into movement) can be linked with each other.

Exercises with the following emphases are especially useful in connection with movement and thought:

- Endurance
- Ability to move hands / fingers and feet / toes, fine motorics
- Coordination
  - Balance
  - Fitting in with partner and group
  - Adapting to equipment
  - Adapting to (changing) situations (Adaptability)
  - Perception
- Reaction speed.

Occasionally, events and special activities provide an opportunity to try out such abilities, e.g. gymnastics at a dizzying height, piling up crates or climbing a rock or climbing a facade. Regular training, however, seldom takes place on such occasions, which are usually used as attractions at a festival rather than a regular hobby. Regular training generally takes place at the weekly training sessions.

Often this particularly involves variations which train several of the above mentioned fields in combination.

3.3 Social Contacts and Their Link with Mental and Physical Fitness

The positive effects of exercise on thinking have already been described in detail. The physiological changes are independent of whether the exercises are carried out alone or as part of a group. For general well being, however, the social context is of considerable significance. Apart from that, mental activity is increased when physical activity takes place in a group.

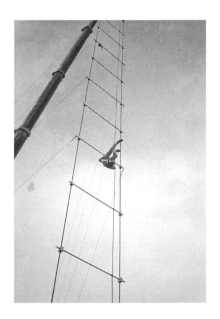
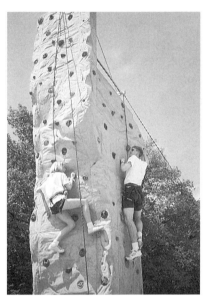
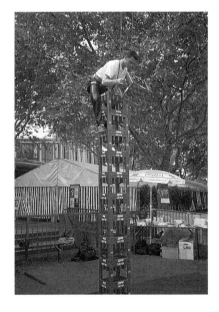

Taking part in gymnastics and sport in a club means being part of a community. Social contacts are encouraged and the animation to further activities above and beyond pure exercise is almost an automatic side effect. Anyone involved in a club is hardly likely to be exposed to the "risk factor mental laziness".

The involvement in a wide range of activities, dealing with other people – getting annoyed at each other as well as being glad together – prevents mental rigidity, makes sure the obstinacy of age does not even have a chance to develop and encourages openness and flexibility, in the literal sense as well.

4 The Brain

4.1 The Human Control Centre

The brain is the human's most important organ, the control centre for all thinking, planning and action. This is where stimuli from the environment are registered. This is where they are processed. And from here the commands for all actions are formulated. The brain makes us conscious of information from the environment and allows us to think about it. Despite huge advances in brain research, because of the complexity of this organ, scientists have still not explored every spiral and furrow.

In recent years, however, one important thing has come to light: The previous common assumption that as one grows older, brain cells (neurons) die, has been proven wrong. On the basis of this false assumption it had been accepted that mental fitness has to decrease at an advanced age. Today, however, it is known that in a healthy person no brain cells die before the age of 70. It is not so much the number of nerve cells that are important for the proper functioning of information processing, but rather the number of connections between them (synapses). The number of these synapses is dependent on training. This means that a lack of stimuli or training does not cause brain cells to die off, but rather it causes the synapses to degenerate.

The nerve cells (neurons) are the smallest independent units of the brain. As far as is currently known, the average person has about 300 billion neurons, which are responsible for the exchange of information and for learning.

The neurons consist of a cell body and a cell core.

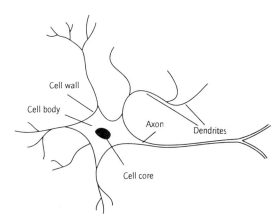

Figure 4:
Nerve cells (neurons) with dendrites and axons

Cell wall

Cell body

Axon

Dendrites

Cell core

They absorb information through numerous tentacles (dendrites). A nerve cell extension or conduit (axon) passes on this information. At its end, it branches out and establishes links (synapses) with other cells, making contact with them. The nerve cells communicate with each other by releasing chemical messenger substances (neurotransmitters). A single nerve cell can develop between 1,000 and 10,000 such synapses and thus create direct connections between cells. The number of these direct connections is a major determinant of how quickly information is passed on. If only a few synapses exist – in the case of a mentally untrained person – more time will be needed to pass on information. Such a person is considered by others to be "slow".

In chapter 3 "Brain Training and Exercise" we have already shown that exercise can have a positive effect on the number of synapses.

4.2 The Left and Right Halves of the Brain

If we look at the brain from above we can recognise the division of the cerebrum in a left and a right half. In the course of the development of the human brain, the two halves have worked out a kind of division of labour among themselves. They have become specialised.

Thus in right handed people the left half is mainly responsible for all logical - analytical thinking, for language and writing, numbers and arithmetic etc. Here things are consciously carried out one after the other.

The right half, on the other hand, is mainly artistically creative. It considers things as a whole, intuitively, to a large extent unconsciously. Here pictures and symbols are processed. It picks up music, mimicry, body language etc. Automated activities originate here.

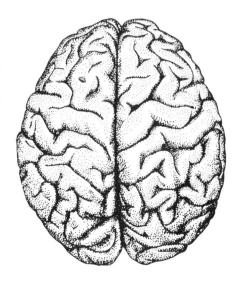

Figure 5:
The human brain seen from above.

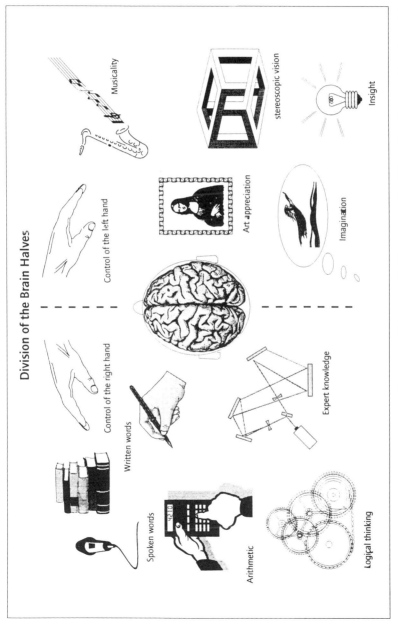

Figure 6: Division of the Brain Halves (created by Bettina M. Jasper with Cliparts from Corel Draw, Corel Corporation, Canada)

There is a constant exchange of information between the two. In this way, behavioural unity is ensured.

During movement, both brain halves are often in use. For example, if the trainer explains the exercise orally, the left half of the brain picks up and processes the information. If this is accompanied by body language, if an expression of movement is also perceived, or if there is musical accompaniment etc., then the right half of the brain is also involved. Finally, the better an exercise has been learnt, the more it happens automatically, the more the left half moves into the background and the right half determines events. In addition, the cerebellum takes over a part of the tasks, namely control over the unconscious motoric functions.

4.3 Facts and Figures

- On average the human brain weighs between 1,200 and 1,500 g. The male brain weighs c. 1,500 g, the female brain weighs c. 1,250.
- In relationship to total body weight a human has a very large brain. The human relationship body weight: brain weight is 50 : 1; a crocodile, for example, has a relationship of 13,000 : 1.
- Every day c. 1,000 litres of blood flow through the human brain. It needs c. 70 litres of oxygen daily. Daily sugar (glucose) consumption is about 100 g, which is about half of the total glucose consumption of the entire body.
- The brain has an average of 300 billion nerve cells (neurons). In spite of differing brain weights, men and women have the same number of brain cells.
- Each of these nerve cells can develop between 1,000 and 10,000 synapses. Thus an average of 300 to 2,000 billion synapses can be calculated. The number of synapses changes in the course of one's life and is dependent on their use.
- In a healthy person the number of nerve cells does not decrease before the age of 70, and after that the decrease is also minimal.
- Blood circulation in the brain is higher in men than in women.
- Stimuli can be passed on at a speed of up to 400 km/h.
- The left brain half (of right handed people) is logical-analytical, the right half is artistic-creative. They cooperate closely with each other.
- The two halves are linked by the so-called beam which consists of more than 200 million nerve fibres.

5 What Needs to Be Trained?

5.1 Crystallised and Liquid Intelligence

In daily life it quickly becomes obvious which aspects of brain performance are causing us problems. Usually, we have little difficulty remembering things we stored in our memory long ago and which are important to us. Thus a healthy person never forgets his or her own name, nor the names of people important in his or her life. Remembering our own address or birthday also requires no great effort. It takes a little more effort to remember what we had for lunch yesterday. We can answer the question: How much is 4 x 7? without a major arithmetical operation because our times table is firmly implanted. But we have to do some serious thinking if 4 is to be divided by 1.5 - after all, here the answer is not quite so simple. If someone asks us to complete the phrase "Nothing ventured ...", we usually reply "nothing gained" without hesitating. Yet if we are asked to repeat the sentence before last spoken by the other person, that is often difficult.

In other words: We can generally immediately recall knowledge and experience gained over many years, memorised and repeatedly used without thinking about it much. Information stored in our memory in this way is called "crystalline intelligence". This information is firmly implanted in our brain. This crystalline or crystallised intelligence is less susceptible to disruption and is frequently very distinct at an advanced age. It allows us to make use of accumulated knowledge and decades of experience.

What causes most difficulty in daily life is "fluid intelligence". It comes into play when we have to cope with situations in which we cannot rely on stored knowledge and experience. Fluid intelligence is required when current problems have to be solved where we cannot apply earlier experiences. Orientation in traffic is affected in the same way as storing new information: How do you programme the new videorecorder, what did the technician say this morning?

People call this short term memory, that does not always function as we would wish it. Today science calls this "short term storage capacity", as it is not our actual memory that is involved here but in particular the processing and short term retention of information. This short term storage capacity is reduced noticeably by a lack of training and older people often have problems with it when they do not deliberately stimulate it.

5.2 Information Processing

Figure 7 shows the complex system of human information processing.

Stimuli from the environment are picked up by the senses and conducted into the short term storage area. This processes the information for a few seconds and either transforms it into actions or stores it in the memory.

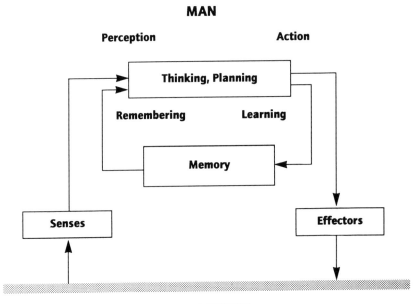

Figure 7: Model of information processing (cf.: Lehrl, Siegfried / Fischer, Bernd / Lehrl, Maria; Series Gehirntraining: Gejo-Leitfaden. Ein Überblick über Gehirn-Jogging - Grundlagen und Anwendungen, Vless Verlag, Ebersberg, 1990, page 21)

Every piece of information which is meant to be consciously available to us must be present in the short term storage area from whence it can be called up from memory when required. The short term storage area takes responsibility for thinking and planning and makes decisions. It is a kind of working memory of the brain, the memory, the archive or comparable with the hard disc of a computer. The short term storage area is considered the centre of fluid intelligence, while the centre of crystallised intelligence is located in the memory.

In other words, every piece of information has two possibilities after processing in the short term storage area: either it is immediately transformed into action via the so-called effectors *(Latin term in stimulus physiology for gland, muscle or organ systems which react actively to stimuli picked up and passed on)* and is thus no longer relevant for us, or it is stored in our memory to be called up again later.

In a gymnastics and sport session both situations can occur. Brief instructions and tasks are registered by the participants and immediately transformed into movement, i.e. action, and usually do not need to be stored in their memories. If, however, they are learning a game that they will further develop and train in the next session, then they need to store the rules in their memories and to remember them as completely as possible next time. Retention is also important when practising demonstrations etc.

5.3 Training Approaches and Methods

The short term storage area is the area which – especially as we get older – needs to be intensively trained.

There are a variety of possibilities and methods to train the brain. First of all it always makes sense to keep fit in the context of general, unspecific mental activation. This can be done by having a range of hobbies and interests. Reading is a good way to keep mentally flexible. Social games are also not just a way to pass the time but additionally an activating factor. Many of these activities provide an opportunity to join with other people and maintain a sense of community and sociability. Gymnastics and sport in particular are often a welcome diversion in daily life.

Numerous methods of training mental abilities have been developed especially in recent years. Each has a different emphasis, trains with different approaches. What the individual chooses depends on his or her objectives. Concentration training, learning techniques and strategies, association exercises etc. are offered just as are creativity training or mnemonic techniques whose application can lead to absolute performance and records or even to world memory championships. Depending on your interests and tendencies, you can choose and practise one or the other. Many methods complement each other and it makes sense to combine them. It is important, however, that first the basic functions of the brain are trained. When the basic functions have been trained and the short term storage area capacity is thus satisfactory, the demands of daily life can be well coped with and it is easier to learn and practise special techniques that are based on them.

With regard to the ability to remember things and the problems this causes in daily life, two methods in particular are common, both involving an abundance of training material: Memory Training and so-called Brain Jogging.

Deliberate training – usually in a casual atmosphere – is provided in particular by Dr. med. Franziska Stengel's "Memory Training" which has long been used in working with the elderly. Various categories of games, puzzles and concentration exercises are used to demand and encourage mental alertness. Fun and enjoyment are major factors here. Often well known sayings are used as training material, but creativity and imagination are also called for and association – developing links between thoughts – is also practised. Finding the right word is given high priority in these exercises. Memory training frequently provides an opportunity to use knowledge acquired some time ago, for example when participants are required to find or guess a single term for certain groups of words or which term does not match the others. Memory training requires much crystallised intelligence which is often very advanced in elderly people.

The method known as Brain Jogging, which has also made a name for itself under the title "Fischer-Lehrl Method" (after its creators), has another approach. In scientific terms it is a "Mental Activation Training" (MAT), also called "Integrative Brain Performance Training" (IBPT). It involves deliberate brain performance training in order to create an optimum starting basis for mental fitness within a short time – c. five to ten minutes. Various exercises are used to mainly train the short term storage area capacity. In the basic exercises numbers, letters and symbols without meaning are used. In this way the emphasis is on mechanical training and there is no distraction through thinking about the meaning. In Brain Jogging, Mental Activation Training or Integrative Brain Performance Training the emphasis is on training the basic functions of the brain. In this way a starting point is created with which complementary methods can later be combined. Brain Jogging is thus more or less a warming up for mental activity that follows – just like the warm up before every sporting activity.

6 Basic Functions of the Brain

Here we will describe five basic functions of the brain – also known as informational psychological basic factors:

- Speed of information processing
- Attention span (also: presence)
- Basic learning speed (also: short term retention)
- Memory capacity
- Endurance ability

The first two are the most important in the whole system as together they form – as a product – the short term storage area capacity which – as we mentioned already in the previous section "Training approaches and methods" – needs to be specially trained.

Let us now discuss what is meant in each case and how these functions can be trained.

6.1 Speed of Information Processing

The speed of information processing indicates the length of time taken to perceive information or stimuli from the environment via the senses, to process them in the short term storage area – i.e. to think about them, and finally, after a decision, to react, i.e. to act on them.

In daily life this basic function/factor of the brain is especially required in traffic. We walk or drive towards traffic lights. The lights go red. We perceive the red light (stimulus from the environment) with our eyes (senses), process the information in our short term storage area (briefly think about the significance), quickly call up the information stored in our memory about red lights, link this with our current perception and finally transform the result of this thinking, the decision - the necessity to stop – into action and either come to a standstill ourselves or brake our vehicle. Similarly complicated processes take place at an amazing speed in every training session in which we are constantly required to combine current pieces of information and act accordingly.

Typical basic exercises for training information processing speed are so-called crossing out exercises. In line with constantly changing examples and patterns, certain combinations of numbers, letters or symbols must be recognised quickly and crossed out. This must be done very quickly, at the risk of missing out individual figures.

After going through quickly the first time, go through the crossed out figures, add them up and note the sum at the end of a column or line. Now follows a second look to check the results. If you really did it quickly the first time, you are bound to find a number of figures you missed. Here are some examples:

Example 1 - Crossing Out Exercise

Quickly go through the columns below from top to bottom. Cross out any figures that are the same which are ordered in the way shown at the top:

Column 1	Column 2	Column 3	Column 4	Column 5
40	37	272	DKJ	KTEK
33	14	7	RLLA	RKKU
59	45	151	PDXE	LMEZ
22	90	905	EOÜT	STIP

Column 1	Column 2	Column 3	Column 4	Column 5
48	18	341	ASTT	SNBM
00	84	759	RTTE	EPÜE
58	29	585	OPFG	TEER
72	42	028	GGSI	XVUK
33	23	371	AQLM	ASLA
99	71	727	RXDD	RAAI
17	55	508	WDDÖ	TUBM
32	50	473	ZUTF	OZMU
55	21	502	VBEU	QERQ
61	13	010	MURR	PQQU
94	44	642	CRRE	ZUITN
66	39	252	HBNA	WDRE
38	92	585	AKLL	DURD
72	47	838	BLLE	FDDL
55	36	901	TBGH	BOKS
17	63	364	UOAL	SFVB
44	52	565	ZUBB	NCCS
80	17	142	ABBI	UOTR

Example 2 - Crossing Out Exercise

Quickly go through the following lines from left to right. In each line cross out the combination of figures shown above each line:

482
45984589467894875119849684634824857487802482458749687936923482

GAN
FGKJGFGFQNALHGANAUEÖRFÖLMEWENGANZSDÖTZQIGAMTGBUMGAN

tz
kleflkmlkjklrtztjglkgjtztzkjlkfzkzfzmasvebhnfekznartzkrtzkjaögafghrgfbnfgrta

♣♦
♚≺⑤♠♥➤➜❾♛❢♣♦⋏❸≻❷♠♥⟴⋏❸≻❷♠♣♦♥⟴⟴❾❽❷♠♣♦♥⟴Ⅴ

Such exercises are usually carried out in courses or on one's own using worksheets, i.e. at a table and not while in movement. Some elements, however, can be linked with exercises in the gym and incorporated in training sessions in another form. Examples of this can be found in the chapter "Brain Training During Practical Sports Lessons" (page49).

6.2 Attention Span (Also: Presence Span)

The attention span, also frequently referred to as presence, is the second basic function / factor. It describes the length of time in which a piece of information is directly and consciously available to us, in which it is present for us. The attention span is only a few seconds, on average 5.4 seconds, and can be extended to up to 7 seconds with appropriate training.

In daily life this function is important when information that need not remain in memory has to be briefly stored, for example when crossing the street. Before you cross the street you look first left, then right (in countries with righthand drive first right, then left). Sometimes your glance remains briefly fixed to the right – perhaps because you feel you have seen something interesting – and when you then really want to cross the street, you have to look left again because you no longer know if the street was clear in this direction.

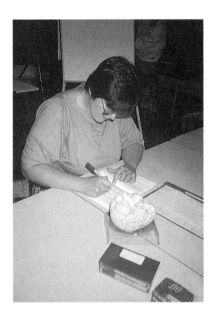

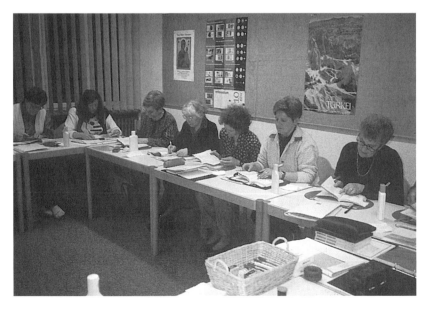

In the gymnastics session the trainer explains an exercise briefly. You follow attentively, but during the second part of the explanatory sentence you are so busy with understanding that by the end of the short description, you have already forgotten the first part of the exercise.

Typical basic exercises for training presence are for example repeating or writing down letters or numbers after seeing or hearing them once. It is very important here not to use tricks or strategies for better retention. It is not the correct result that is important here but the training – i.e. the lengthening – of the attention span. Numbers or figures are called out roughly every second and should be immediately repeated out loud or written down – without repeating them mentally or using rhythmical groups or logical systems to memorise them. Exercises with playing cards that have numbers or letters printed on them also work this way.

Example 1 - Card Exercise

Take such a card game, briefly uncover a card every second and put it away out of sight. First try it with four or five cards. Immediately afterwards write down the sequence and check if you have it right. You will quickly discover that the amount you can retain and immediately recall in this way is limited. Four or five figures can usually be retained quite easily, but then it gets difficult. If you keep to the pace of one per second, at the limit of your attention span you will recall a maximum of seven figures.

Example 2 - Repeating Figures

Look at the sequence of figures in one of the lines on the left for five seconds and cover them up. Immediately write the figures – if possible in the same order - in the empty spaces on the right.

31	5	71	9	36
K	S	T	X	Z
ä	ü	ö	y	e
MUL	SIR	PEM	NAX	ZIT
O	✂	☎	✪	☺

Such exercises are generally carried out in courses or in individual training using playing cards or worksheets. Some elements of these exercises can, however, be linked with exercises in the gym and incorporated in training sessions in another form. Examples of this can be found in the chapter "Brain Training During Practical Sports Lessons" (page49).

6.3 Basic Learning Speed (Also: Short Term Retention)

This third basic function / factor is also referred to as "Short term retention". It describes the amount of information which can be stored and called up again in a certain unit of time after it is no longer present, i.e. no longer in the short term storage area. This means that information is initially consciously stored. Afterwards there follows a period of distraction so that the information can enter the memory, and later the recall, consciously making the information available.

In daily life problems with short term retention often manifest themselves as disturbances in our ability to remember things. I write a shopping list and go into town to buy the items on the list. Of course, I leave the list at home. Now I try to recall from memory what I had written down in order to get everything after all. Do I always manage it without forgetting something?
   In training sessions this function is often required - always in those cases when new movement sequences, choreographies, dances, rules etc. must be learned.
   Typical basic exercises consist of a changing number of information units, - numbers, letters, words, symbols ... - which initially have to be consciously stored. After this comes deliberate distraction so that the information in the short term storage area can go into our memory. A conversation in the group can serve as a diversion, or a completely different task such as an arithmetical sum which requires the full attention of the participants. After that the information is recalled and made available, i.e. written down, spoken or reproduced in action.

Example 1

Memorise the following numbers and then cover them up. Now count backwards from 100 by subtracting 4 each time - i.e. 100, 96, 92 ... Then write down all the numbers you can still remember.

6 - 38 - 72 - 14 - 25 - 47 - 95

Example 2

Memorise the syllables in the box on the left and then cover them up (the box on the right remains covered the whole time). Divide 3,152 by 14 in your head to three spaces after the decimal point. Now uncover the box on the right and cross out the syllables you did not see on the left.

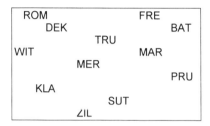 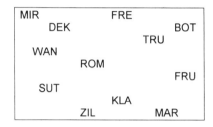

Such exercises are generally carried out in courses or in individual training using playing cards or worksheets. Some elements of these exercises can, however, be linked with exercises in the gym and incorporated in training sessions in another form. Examples of this can be found in the chapter "Brain Training During Practical Sports Lessons" (page49)

6.4 Memory Capacity and Endurance Ability

The fourth basic function / factor is memory capacity. It corresponds to the total amount of information stored in the memory. This varies greatly from one invididual to the next and cannot be measured in an acceptable time frame. It is therefore unknown to date just how great the individual differences are. There are great differences in knowledge but this can not be equated with memory capacity because the system used to store information plays a major role here. This in turn is dependent to a great deal on the short term storage area capacity. Special exercises for deliberate training of memory capacity are unknown at this time.

Endurance ability is considered the fifth basic factor. It cannot be extrapolated from the other basic factors and is highly dependent on motivation. Here too, there are no known examples of special training.

6.5 Combined Tasks and Advanced Training

The training examples described so far can be clearly linked to the individual basic functions. They are all typical basic exercises. The material provides little challenge to the senses and the tasks can be solved without any advance information and independent of knowledge and education.

In addition to these basic exercises there are so-called advanced exercises. Here knowledge and education can be incorporated to a certain extent. Logical thinking is also necessary. The advanced exercises are often considered more interesting than the basic exercises. Nevertheless, it is recommended that initially the basic exercises be carried out regularly, for only through these is it possible to precisely address each basic function. By doing balanced basic training you provide a good basis for handling the tasks of the advanced programme more quickly and more easily.

Advanced exercises usually address a combination of basic functions, when for example new information is combined with knowledge, that is with already existent memory content which is recalled. A typical example are so-called scrambled letters. The idea is to re-sort arbitrarily ordered letters so that words with a meaning are created, whereby no letter may be removed or added.

Example: LANOITANRETNI = INTERNATIONAL

Only someone who has heard the word "international" before and stored it in their memory has even a chance of solving the puzzle. The initially apparently unconnected letters have to be combined again and again in the short term storage area and compared with words which are retrieved from memory into the short term storage area and thus made available to us.

The successful processing of such combined and advanced exercises usually leads to a result or one or more solutions. The feeling of success in this case is perhaps greater for some than in the basic exercises in which there is often no tangible result which confirms one's achievement. Seen the other way, however, the unsuccessful search for a solution can reduce training motivation.

The solutions of the advanced exercises tend to remain in our memory for a long time. For this reason, work with such training materials can only be repeated after long pauses. A repetition of basic exercises after a short period of time is, on the other hand, not a problem at all in most cases.

In consideration of the above mentioned aspects, it is advisable in regular training to complement daily basic training, which uses materials that do not challenge the senses a great deal, with a variety of interesting tasks from the advanced programme and thus to address a combination of various basic functions.

Examples of such combined exercises for mental training can be found in the Appendix for use in the Brain Fitness Circuit. These and similar worksheets provide material not only for training mental fitness, but – with a little imagination and experience – can be combined with movement by incorporating only minor changes. When the individual elements are put on posters or transformed using polystyrene letters and numbers, foam circles and triangles, coloured cloth etc., such worksheets can take on a completely new dimension in the gym.

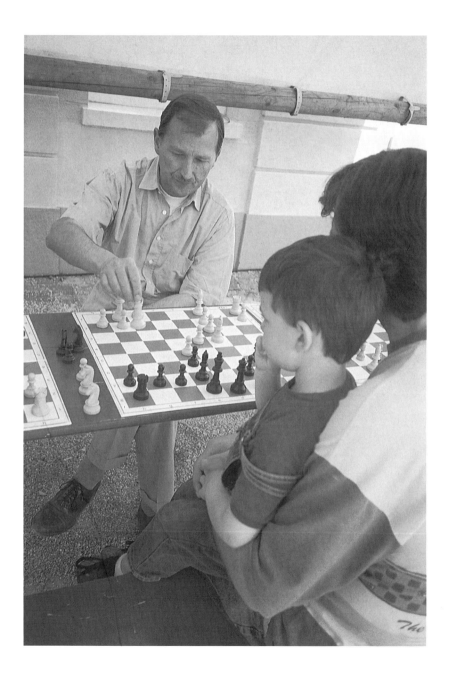

7 Brain Training During Practical Sports Lessons

7.1 General Considerations

In previous chapters we have indicated several times that club training sessions are a good opportunity to also train the brain. First of all – as already mentioned – general sports activity in a group can already be seen as mental activation in itself. Of course the emphasis remains on the physical training aspect. But just\as physical activity in a group always has social aspects as well, it is also accepted that it has an effect on mental fitness.

Brain training in clubs does not mean that in future an extra slot has to be planned in the training programme. The idea is not to develop a completely new type of training.

Rather, we want to demonstrate that many elements of traditional training, in addition to many other positive effects, can also aid training of the brain. Sometimes the exercises carried out automatically contain forms of brain training - the trainer just does not know it or has not consciously used them to train the brain. Sometimes small but decisive changes can be made to familiar exercises and games which also make them effective in training mental fitness. Occasionally, minor changes to the training sequence can have a major effect. For example, it can be helpful to move a fine motoric exercise from the end of the session to the beginning of a phase in which a new dance is to be learnt. Finger exercises increase the blood flow to the brain and thus make it easier for the participants to digest the new complicated information when learning the dance.

A number of such exercises which affect the brain will be shown on the following pages. They are intended to encourage trainers to reconsider their own exercise programmes in this light, to carry out any necessary minor changes and above all to emphasise the positive effects of particular exercises on mind and memory. Comprehensively informing participants about the background and function of individual exercises is a decisive factor for judging the quality of the exercises. With increasing health consciousness and in particular the growing fear of reduced brain performance as one ages, it is becoming increasingly important to give adult club members in-depth information.

7.2 Examples of Exercises and Games

The examples given here should not be incorporated as a block in the training session but should be spread throughout the session.

In the chapter "Brain Training and Exercise", the main areas were shown in which it is useful to link exercise and thinking. The following exercises cannot always be attributed to a certain area but frequently address and train several aspects in combination. For this reason they are not divided into the various motoric functions to be addressed or categorised in any other way. The order they are given in therefore does not indicate any kind of system.

To help allot the suggestions to particular situations, the examples have been given three distinct symbols:

 Exercises and games which require room to move – in some cases a hall.

 Exercises and games which can be carried out in a closed space.

 Exercises and games which can be carried out quickly during meetings, at social events, on trips or in similar situations as an "active break".

Note:
When it is a matter of speed, according to the kind of group, difficulties should be added so that it is not the speed which determines the game but mainly abilities controlled by the brain. For example balancing something on one's head, rolling a tyre alongside oneself, carrying cottonwool in the palm of one's hand etc.

Many kinds of games where music is stopped not only train endurance but additionally require increased attentiveness as well as quick reactions and decisions and also adaptation to partners, the group and the music. With regard to improved blood circulation in the brain (see motoric Homunculus, page22) it is a good idea to have the group sing along.

 ### *Who Stood Where?*

Task: The group forms a square. If there are 12 people each side consists of four, if there are 25 each side consists of five etc. If the numbers do not allow this, a rectangle is formed. Each person briefly memorises the exact composition of the group. Who is standing next to whom? Who is standing opposite? ... As soon as the music starts, the group moves freely to the music. When it stops, everyone gets back to the original position as quickly as possible.

Variation 1: As above, but after the music the square or rectangle should be reassembled 90° or 180° to the left or right.

Variation 2: As above, but each time the new formation is moved one position to the left or right.

Variation 3: As above, but the pattern is different – a polygon, a star ... It can also be a letter or a number.

Variation 4: As above, but the formation is a mirror image of the original formation (best done with a line through the middle as a mirror axis).

Variation 5: As above, but before the music phase it is agreed which two persons will swap places in the new formation. In experienced groups a number of people can change places.

Find the Shape!

Task: Everyone moves freely to the music. When the music stops, they look for a marking or an object in the room which is round (e.g. a tyre lying on the floor, centre marking on a playing field ...) or square (e.g. little box, foam shapes, spread out newspapers ...) – depending on what the trainer shows – and go to it as quickly as possible.

Variation 1: The music consists of instrumental and sung passages. A break during an instrumental means look for round shapes, during singing it means look for squares.

Variation 2: Other shapes are added, e.g. triangle, straight line, curve, star ...

Variation 3: Instead of shapes, colours are run to - for blue a blue mat, for green a green line ...

Material: Boards with a circle, square, triangle and other shapes or else easily recognisable objects which can be shown.

 ### *Atom Game*

Task: Everyone moves freely to the music. When the music stops, a number is called out or shown. If it is e.g. a "4", the participants move as quickly as possible to create "atoms" consisting of four persons. When all are ready, the music starts again.

Variation 1: When the music stops, the trainer holds up a big word sign. The number of letters is to be recognised as quickly as possible and transformed into groups of the corresponding number of persons. If the word "house" is on the sign, groups of five persons should be formed. If it says "railway", groups of seven are required. It is more difficult if the word is merely called out, for then everyone has to imagine the word written down and count the letters.

Variation 2: A number between 1 and 12 is chosen. This number represents a month, e.g. 5 for May or 12 for December. Only those born in this month form a group. Everyone else continues to move about the room and sing along with the melody.

Variation 3: When the music stops, a particular characteristic is named, according to which the participants must group themselves, e.g. hair colour – all blondes join together, all brunettes, all with grey hair etc. – or shoe size – then all with shoe size 39 form a group, all with 38 another etc.

Ground Contact

Task: Everyone moves freely about the room to music or singing, and watches the trainer all the time. When she or he indicates a number – either on a board, by showing fingers or calling it out   the participants must touch the ground with a corresponding number of parts of their bodies. If the number is "5" for example, they could touch the ground with two feet and three fingers, i.e. a total of five parts of the body. Other possibilities might be with their bottom and four toes or bottom, two feet and two palms etc. When everyone has achieved the right ground contact the movement starts again.

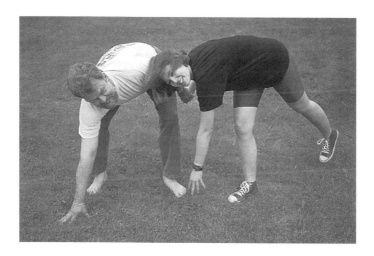

Variation 1: The players do not walk or run around the room individually but in pairs holding hands. Each pair has to jointly fulfill the required number of ground contacts. If for example "2" is called out, A and B can each stand on one leg, so that between them they have two ground contacts.

Variation 2: Like Variation 1, but A and B can only communicate non-verbally.

 ### *Robots*

Task: The participants form pairs, with one person standing behind the other. One person is a "robot" which is steered by the other person. Both move around the room freely, with the robot following the signals of the other. It is important that the robots only take small and slow steps. Tapping both shoulders at once means straight ahead, tapping on the left or right shoulder means a 90° turn – i.e. a right angle – in the appropriate direction. Placing hands on both shoulders means "stop". Note: Of course the other pairs in the room must be taken into consideration and the robot must be carefully directed through the "traffic".

After a brief period the partners swap roles.

Variation 1: As above, but the robots shut their eyes.

Variation 2: As above, but to ensure safe movement through the room, the steerer leaves his or her hands on the shoulders of the robot and makes the signals with a brief exertion of pressure.

Variation 3: Groups of three are formed. Two robots are steered by one person. At the start the two "motorscooters" stand back to back. The idea is to move them both so that at the end they stand facing each other. If a robot meets an obstacle it stays there until it is released by the person steering.

This version is only possible with a very mobile group. The steerer in particular must move around constantly. The exercise is only possible outside or in a large room.

Number Running

Task: Large signs with numbers from 1 to X are mixed up and stuck to the walls all around the room. The number of signs depends on the size of the room and the group. For a group of 15 for example the numbers 1 to 15 can be used. Each participant begins with a number between 1 and 15. Mary begins at "1", Jim at "2", Louise at "3" etc. Beginning at their starting number, each person runs to the numbers that follow. That means that Louise starts at "3" and then runs to "4", then to "5" etc. When she reaches "15" she then continues with "1" and has only reached her goal when she has run to "2".

As evidence that everyone has run to all numbers in the correct order, each person writes their initial and the number of each point for them on the sign with the pen that has been placed there. Thus Louise writes "L.1" at sign 3,; at sign 4 she writes "L.2", while Jim writes "J.3" at sign 4. Is that clear? Or has anyone got the number sequence mixed up?

Material: Large number signs (at least DIN A 4), cellotape, a pen for each sign (best if tied with string and attached to the sign so no one takes it with them).

Crossing Out Numbers

Task: The group is divided into teams of three or four persons. Each team lines up. At the other end of the room is a large poster with numbers for each team. On it are numbers from 1 to X, e.g. to 22 (see number poster in Appendix, page127), completely mixed up. There are small and large numbers in different scripts in different sized spaces. The numbers must be crossed out by each team in ascending order. The team members individually run to the turning point, look for the next number, cross it out, run back and give the pen to the next team member.

Material: A number poster for each team (size at least DIN A 4). Depending on the size of the room and the poster it may be a good idea to fix a covering page to the poster (like a calendar) so that those with "eagle eyes" cannot already determine the next number from their waiting position but must really look for the number when they arrive at the turning point.

Note: You can practise for this exercise at home at a desk by crossing out numbers (or letters) on appropriate worksheets.

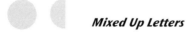

Mixed Up Letters

Task: The trainer thinks of a word that has as many letters as the group has members: e.g. "CONSTITUTION" for 12 people. (With larger groups it is advisable to divide into two or three smaller groups.) Accordingly he or she prepares twelve sheets of paper or cardboard with one letter each on them. The signs should be at least DIN A 5 in size so that they can be read by everyone at a considerable distance.

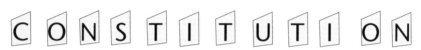

Each participant receives one sign which is initially not visible to the others. Only when the trainer gives the signal does the group begin to move around the room. Each person carries their sign visibly in front of themselves.

Whilst walking or running around the room the participants get an overview of which letters are available. Then they attempt to group themselves in such a way as to create a word that has meaning, in which all letters are used. If anyone thinks they have recognised part of the word, they can try to link up with the people who have the letters next to them. For example if someone with an "O" thinks the word might contain "ION", then they must try to link up with "I" and "N". This in turn could put other group members on the right track and they might experiment further, e.g. putting "STITUT" next to it etc.

It is important that all keep to the agreement not to communicate verbally. Sign language, mimicry and gestures are allowed. Standing still during the game is strictly forbidden. Everything takes place in a moving environment.

If the group does not come closer to the solution on its own the trainer should give small clues after a certain time, for example the first letter (if necessary also the second, third ... letter) or a tip about the subject – legal term, it has something to do with a nation etc.

Variation 1: Instead of letters, words are handed out, which the participants must join into a sensible sentence.

Variation 2: Long words or short sentences are divided into syllables and each sign shows a syllable instead of a letter in the original version.

Variation 3: Instead of signs with letters, picture cards are handed out. With these the participants create nouns made of word combinations and keep forming new pairs. Someone with a picture of RAIN joins a person with a picture of a BOW (RAIN-BOW). At every signal from the trainer the pairs split up and look for new partnerships. Thus RAIN could join up with HAT (RAIN-HAT), while BOW pairs off with MAN (BOW-MAN).

Reaction - Skill - Team

Task: Teams of 4-5 people line up. The team members number off. Each team receives a raquet (badminton, beach tennis, table tennis or similar) and a ball. The ball is transported on the raquet around the team and is not allowed to fall. If it falls, the participant has to go back to the starting position and begin again. The team members do not have their turn in sequence, instead the trainer calls out a number, and the corresponding team member has their turn. Thus from each team the person with the number 3 might run (see illustration), then the person with the number 5 etc.

Raquet and ball always have to be collected from their basic position and brought back again at the end. Whoever is back at their position first scores a point for their team.

Variation 1: As above, but each time with a different kind of movement – sideways, backwards, crouched, bent over ...

Variation 2: As above, but in each round the number and the starting position changes. All players move along one space.

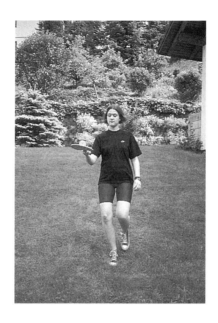

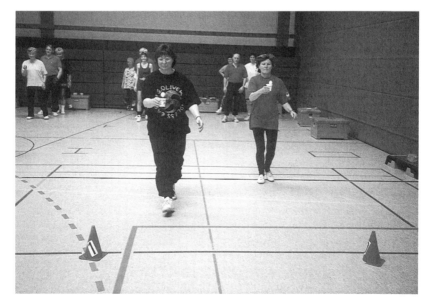

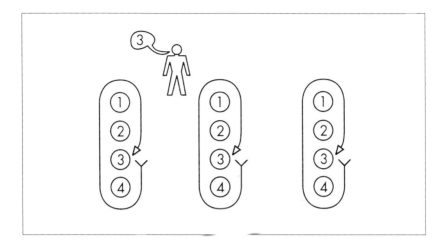

Figure 8: Reaction - Skill - Team (created by Bettina M. Jasper with Cliparts from Corel Draw, Corel Corporation, Canada)

 Rainmaker

Situation: The trainer tells the group a story in which, after a long dry spell, everyone is longing for rain. Because the rain will not come of its own accord, together the group copies the sounds which are heard when rain slowly builds up, gradually gets harder and harder until it is absolutely pouring, and then slowly eases and finally stops completely.

Task: The sounds are created in this way: Everyone sits or stands in a circle. The trainer stands in the middle of the circle and shows the movements, turning slowly and looking at the participants one by one. Everyone carries out the movement until another movement is called for. In every round a new movement is required: rubbing the palms of the hands together, snapping the fingers, slapping the thighs, stamping the feet, slapping the thighs, snapping the fingers, rubbing the palms of the hands together.

Variation: As above, but with closed eyes. Each time the sound made by the neighbour on the left is copied and thus passed on.

Tapping the Fingers

Task: All tap hard with their fingertips on a hard surface – hall floor, wall, bench, table ...

Variation 1: As above, but every tap is counted. Who will reach 100 first?

Variation 2: As above, but the group communicates non-verbally and finally finds a common rhythm.

Variation 3: As above, but each time the trainer announces or shows which fingers are to be used for tapping.

 Arm Vibrator

Task: The arms are held up. In this position the participants must turn their wrists as quickly as possible (as if a screw had to be screwed into the ceiling very quickly).

Note: This exercise can increase the blood flow to the brain by c. 30 %!

 Cork Vice

Task: Who can hold the most corks between their fingers and keep this position for at least 30 seconds?

Variation 1: As above, but the corks can only be picked up by the hand between whose fingers they are to held. The other hand is not allowed to assist.

Variation 2: As above, but the team members join in pairs. Now the corks must be placed between the fingers whilst moving about. Whoever remains standing is out. A carries a container full of corks while B puts them between his or her fingers - then they swap.

Material: Corks (To make it more difficult pingpong balls can be used instead of corks. Much less are needed because not so many can be placed between the fingers as when doing it with corks.)

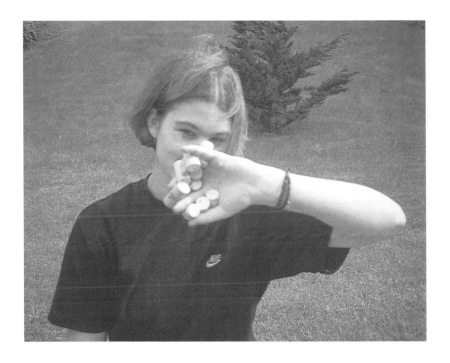

Bumpers

Task: The participants lead each other through the room in alternating pairs (A stands opposite B), in each case with corks as "bumpers" between the index fingertips of both hands - moving forewards, backwards, sideways, with open or closed eyes etc.

Variation: As above, but several corks – theoretically up to ten – must be held between the tips of several fingers. Who can do it standing or even moving, without standing still and without losing the corks?

Material: Corks.

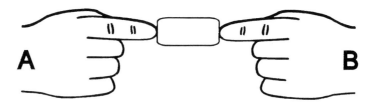

Figure 9 (created by Bettina M. Jasper with Cliparts from Corel Draw, Corel Corporation, Canada)

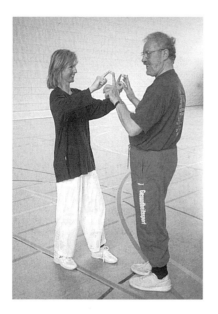 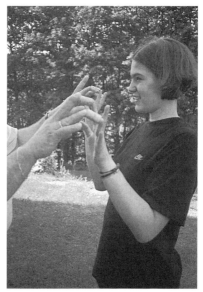

 Finger 1 to 5

Task: The fingers of a hand are brought to the thumb one after the other so that the tips touch each other – index finger, middle finger, ring finger, little finger and back again, when the command is given or at one's own – ever increasing – pace.

*Figure 10
(created by Bettina M. Jasper
with Cliparts from Corel Draw,
Corel Corporation, Canada)*

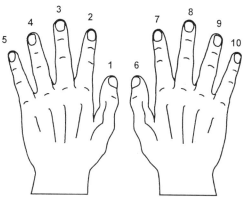

Variation 1. As above, but the fingers of one hand are numbered – Thumb = 1, index finger = 2 etc. to the little finger = 5. Only the numbers are called out and the corresponding fingers of both hands must be moved to the thumb.

Variation 2:
As above, but the numbering begins at the left thumb with 1 and ends at the little finger of the right hand with 10. Now e.g. finger 3 and finger 8 must come together – i.e. both middle fingers – or 1 and 5, 4 and 9 etc.
Are all finger combinations correct?

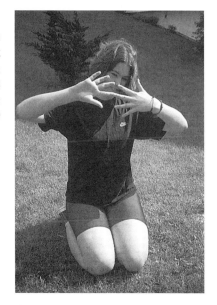

Variation 3:
Groups that have had lots of practice can sit down and include their toes as well and number them too. This expands the spectrum of numbers so e.g. 2 and 18 can come together – the index finger of the left hand and the middle toe of the right foot.

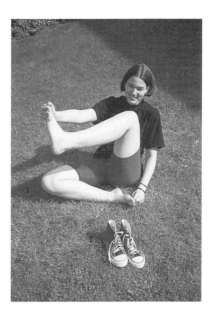

Variation 4: Only the toes are numbered and drawn together.

Variation 5: Like Variation 2, but in pairs. A and B stand opposite each other. A's fingers receive the numbers 1-10, B's receive 11-20. Together they have to find the right combinations as quickly as possible.

 Finger Theatre

Task: Together the group seeks five first names. These are then assigned to the fingers, e.g. thumb = Fred, index finger = Julie, middle finger = Viola, ring finger = Bernie, little finger = Bridget. Now creative imagination is called for. Together the group thinks up a story in which all five names occur in changing order. E.g. "Julie and Fred want to go on vacation. Of course they take their son Bernie and their daughter Viola with them. While Julie and Fred are preparing everything, Viola asks if she can take her friend Bridget. Bridget sits next to Viola at school. Julie is in favour, but Fred says that then Bernie may want to take a friend too. But there is not enough room in the car to take anyone other than Bernie, Viola, Bridget, Julie and Fred ..."The story is written down. When it is then read out all must pay attention, for when a name is read out, the finger theatre becomes active and each time the correct finger has to be held up and moved.

Variation 1: As above, but ten names are allotted instead of five, for the ten fingers – five female for the left hand and five male for the right.

Variation 2: Like variation 1 but without dividing the names into male and female, i.e. the names are all mixed up.

Variation 3: As above, but the story is not written down and read out. Instead, after the names have been chosen and allotted, the group develops the story as each person adds a sentence in which one or more of the chosen names occurs. Not only must the right names and fingers be remembered, but additionally a story with meaning must be created.

Note: The story can of course be created somewhere else and brought along for the finger theatre ready made.

Clasping Hands

Task: The hands are alternately clasped and unclasped. After each unclasping they are then clasped in the neigbouring gap.

Variation 1: In pairs, alternating, A clasps her or his hands and B points at a particular finger of the clasped hands. A must then raise this finger.

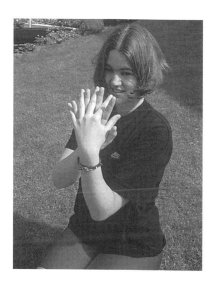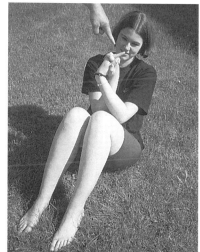

Variation 2: As above, but the finger is named and not pointed at, e.g. "right middle finger" etc.

Variation 3: As above, but before the hands are clasped, the arms are held out and crossed, and the forearms are bent and turned inwards so that the clasped hands are turned through approx. 360°. Now individual fingers are to be raised when named.

 ### *My Hands – Your Hands*

Task: The group sits around a table, stands around a box or similar, or lies in a circle on their stomachs looking into the centre of the circle. Each person crosses hands with their neighbour, i.e. each lays their left hand over and their right hand under the hand of the person sitting or lying next to them. One after the other the pairs of hands on the table or the floor clap. Whose hand is next? Is it mine or yours?

Variation 1: If one hand quickly claps twice, the direction is changed.

Variation 2: Not every hand on the table or floor claps, but only every third hand.

Variation 3: The group sits on the floor in a circle looking into the centre. Instead of the hands the lower legs or feet are crossed. Instead of clapping the feet must now clap or stamp.

 ### *Walking in a Line*

Task: The group is spread around the hall. The objective is to balance on the playing field markings.

Variation 1: The colour of the line must match a piece of one's clothing.

Variation 2: From a fixed point the line is first followed with the eyes (trains the eye muscles!). Only then does one balance on the line.

Variation 3: As in 2, but in pairs. A first follows the line with his or her eyes and then walks the line as accurately as possible with closed eyes. B accompanies A – if necessary holding hands – and makes sure there are no collisions with other pairs.

Variation 4: As in 2, but a certain way of walking must be kept to – on the balls of the feet, bent over, stretching up ...

Drawing Abstract Lines

Task: At the centre of attention is a large poster with a confused tangle of lines. It is hung up for all to see or laid out on the floor. First abstract lines with many curves running between a number and a letter in each case (see example in appendix on page 128) must be identified among the tangle and followed with the eyes. Each member of the group picks a number as start and follows the corresponding line to its end at a letter. He or she memorises the course of the line. After this memorising phase each member chooses a point in the room as a starting point and runs or walks from that point, following the memorised line as exactly as possible. While doing this everyone must keep an eye on the movements of the others to avoid collisions.

Variation 1: As above, but groups of three, four or five persons are formed, each with their own poster of tangled lines. Each player follows the line from one number. In a group of three there are lines 1, 2 and 3, whose ends are marked A to C. In a group of five the lines are 1 to 5 and the ends are A to E. After memorising, the persons 1 to X line up. Opposite them the markers are placed as end points (e.g. clubs or similar). Then 1, 2, 3 ... each follows their own line from the poster. If the line courses are correct, at the finish each end point should be occupied by one person. The better the group works together, the more harmonious the timing will be matched. With much practice the end points will all be reached at the same time.

Variation 2: As above, but each line is occupied by two people, one at the start (number) and one at the end (letter). On the imaginary line they exchange places. If all the line courses are correct, at the finish all start and finish points will be occupied and the group forms a kind of lane.

Obstacle Course

Task: One after the other all members of the group overcome an obstacle course, e.g. first following a line, then crossing a soft surface, after that a bench, then stepping on beer mats followed by balancing on a rope on the ground, after that wading through crates filled with screwed up canvas etc.

Variation: As above, but in groups of three. A and B guide C and give verbal information about the course. C keeps his or her eyes closed. (Only for experienced groups!)

Material: Various pieces of equipment that can be set up as a course with varying surfaces.

Note: It is absolutely important to ensure safety. The course should only be crossed in pairs or threes.

 Beer Mat Course

Task: The trainer lays a course of beer mats around the room. The distance between two mats should be an average step, i.e. approx. 55-65 cm.

The participants move along the course in a line, only stepping on the beer mats.
     The degree of difficulty can be altered by changing the position of the beer mats. If they are laid out in a line, it is more difficult to balance than if they are laid left and right of an imaginary central line.
     The distance between the mats can be altered: large gaps – big steps, small gaps – small steps.

Depending on the group, the course can be crossed alone or helping each other. Thus pairs or groups of three can be formed of which one person crosses the course with one or two others holding her or his hands.

Warning: Choose the length of the gaps in such a way that jumping – and thus the danger of slipping – is avoided! Depending on the floor or ground surface, the beer mats may need to be secured with double-sided adhesive tape to stop them slipping!!!

Variation 1:
The gait for crossing the course is laid down in advance: e.g. only step on the balls of the feet and not extend the foot over the edge of the mats; walk forwards or backwards; walk sideways crossing one's legs.

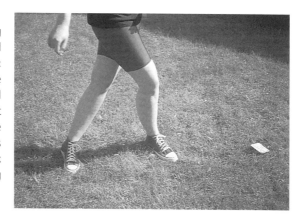

Variation 2: As above, but as an additional difficulty something must be balance across the course without falling: e.g. a beer mat on the head; a beer mat as a tray on which a plastic cup or - more difficult still – a table tennis ball – is carried ...

Variation 3: There is no fixed course, just a certain distance – e.g. from one wall to the other – to be crossed by all participants using beer mats. Each person has three beer mats with which to cross the distance without their feet ever touching the ground directly. I.e. with each foot on a beer mat, the third mat is picked up from behind the person and laid in front repeatedly until the objective is reached.

Targeted Throwing

Task: From a fixed point beer mats are thrown into a tyre lying on the ground or an area marked with tape. Each participant has a certain number, e.g. ten beer mats. How many can they land in the tyre?

Variation 1: As above, but the tyre is not lying on the ground. Instead it is hung above the ground.

Variation 2: As above, but other objects are thrown, e.g. Indiaca balls, rolling balls or similar.

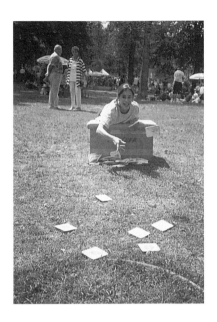

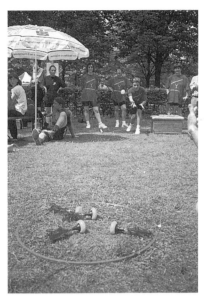

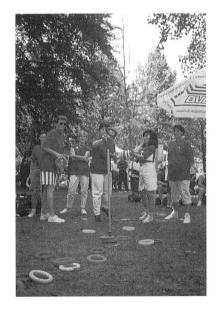

Variation 3:   As above, but more accuracy is required in throwing quoits onto poles.

Material: One tyre to four people and several beer mats or a pole and several quoits.

Tumbler

Task: First lightly and carefully bounce on the Rebounder, then jump.

Variation: As above, but keeping to a prescribed short rhythm, e.g. short - short – short – long – long – long ...

Material: Rebounder.

Note: Depending on the training level of the group this should be done in pairs or groups of three, whereby A and B watch out while C jumps.

Pedalo Riding

Task: Groups of three each stand around a Pedalo. A stands on it, B and C secure A. A tries to move the Pedalo forwards.

Note: Careful when you "brake"!!! Experienced groups as well as children and youths usually need no help and can move the Pedalo forwards on their own.

Material:
One Pedalo per three people.

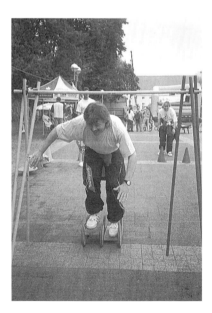

Primaballerina

Task: Groups of three gather round a therapeutic top. A stands on the therapeutic top, B and C secure A. A tries to keep or regain his or her balance in a number of varying positions, after some practice with eyes closed.

Material: One therapeutic top per three people.

Note: If appropriate equipment is available, special designs can be used, e.g. three therapeutic tops linked together by a wooden platform in the middle. By skilfully working together, three people move small balls or marbles around the platform in such a way that they fall into specially cut holes (see photo). Very similar, but used individually, are moving patience games. Here too small balls or marbles must be brought into the centre of a labyrinth. Using appropriate body movement, the balls are moved around the therapeutic top, which in this case is not round but has a special playing tablet mounted on it (see photo).

Standing on Heels

Task: The participants stand on their heels and try to remain in this position for as long as possible. Balancing with one's arms is allowed!

Note: There should be something nearby to hold onto or a wall behind, otherwise do the exercise in pairs! Only to be done with appropriate footwear!

Cup Tennis

Task: Pairs of A and B standing opposite each other hit a table tennis ball to each other using drinking cups or yoghurt containers - the ball is bounced on the floor each time.

Variation 1: As above, but without bouncing the ball.

Variation 2: As above, but with two balls which are both played by A and B at the same time.

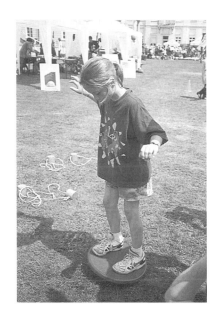

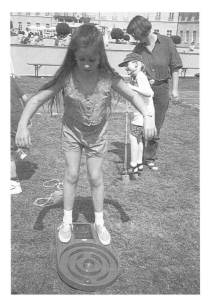

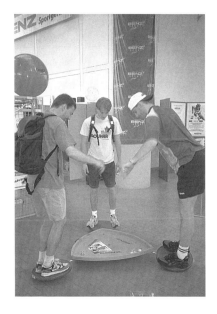

Variation 3: As in 2, but A or B plays both balls at once.

Variation 4:
As above, but moving around.

Variation 5:
As above, but using the hand not normally used – i.e. right handers use the left hand.

Variation 6:
As above, but the ball is played backwards over one's head.

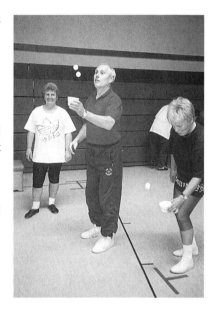

Name Ball

Task: The group stands in a circle. The aim is to learn the names in the group whose members are unknown to each other. In any order the ball is thrown and caught by the group members. A throws the ball to B. When B has caught it, A says his or her name. Now B does the same, throws the ball to C, waits until C has caught it, then says his or her name etc.

Note: This game is often played in a similar way. Not always are the players' names used – instead plants, animals, cities or similar can be named. The important thing about name learning, however, is that initially the order of the actions must be kept to exactly. The brain can only pick up one piece of information at a time! If you throw and name your name at the same time, often a piece of information is not picked up correctly or not stored properly and therefore cannot be called up again later. So: first throw the ball. The catching person moves their fingers when they catch it and thus stimulates the blood circulation to the brain (see motoric homunculus, page 22). Then the brain is well prepared and ready to pick up the new information, the unknown name! After a while the brain needs a new task so it does not automate the processes, so carry on with a variation!

Variation 1: As above, but before throwing, the name of the catcher is called out. Important: Asking before throwing is allowed, otherwise only those people are in the game whose names have been memorised easily.

Variation 2: As above, but after a brief stop the positions in the circle are changed.

Variation 3: As above, but the circle moves, running or walking, around the room.

Variation 4: As in 3, but the group moves around the room out of formation.

Variation 5: As above, but in a group where everyone knows each other well each person gets a new name for the duration of the game – Frank becomes Charles, Mary becomes Louise, and Karen is called Julie from now on. Now who knows who's who?

Material: A ball.

Ball of Words

Task: The group stands in a circle. A player begins, holds a ball of wool and says any word, e.g. "school". Then she or he holds the beginning of the thread tight and throws the ball to someone else in the circle. This person continues with a word that they associate with school, e.g. "holidays", holds tight to a piece of the thread and throws the ball to another person. The catcher says the next association, e.g. "seaside". It could go on with "salt", "pepper", "sneeze", "cold" etc. The game is continued until a net has been formed linking all members of the group to each other.

While forming the net the group should take its time and consciously take in each word and store it in their memories. A good memory is required for the second part of the game. Then the ball of wool has to be rolled up again.

So that the last players are not at an advantage, the group should briefly divert its attention between memorising and rolling up. For this it could e.g. try to move around the room as a net without creating any holes.

Depending on the agility of the group, different gaits can be tried out. Can everyone manage to sit or even lie down at the same time without the net breaking?

After the period of diversion the rolling up starts. The chain of words must be recalled in reverse sequence. The person who said "cold" and is holding the rest of the ball of wool begins. She or he says the word the predecessor said, i.e. "sneeze", and throws the ball to this person who rolls up the thread and meanwhile tries to remember the word before. The next throw is back to "pepper" etc. until finally the ball has been completely rolled up again.

Variation 1: As above, but more tangled. The game goes on until each person has two loops of thread in their hands, i.e. until there are twice as many words involved.

Variation 2: As above, but the words should not be related in any way, but rather just added on arbitrarily. This makes it more difficult to remember them.

Variation 3: As above, but in groups whose members do not know each other's names yet the names are used instead of associations.

Variation 4: As in variations 1 and 3 in combination, i.e. every player has two turns and says their first name in the first round and their last name in the second round.

Variation 5: As in variation 4, but the order of first and last names is not kept to. If someone said their last name in the first round, then this has to be remembered second when rolling up the ball again. With other players the order can also be reversed.

Variation 6: As in the original version, except this time it is not a matter of remembering but of quick processing of information and rapid thinking. Instead of words, letters are called out when the ball is thrown. It is important to choose the letters in such a way that at the end a meaningful word, as long as possible, is created as a joint production. One player begins e.g. with "F" and throws the ball on. The next ones carry on, e.g. with "L", "O", "W",

"E", "R" etc. Thus through good teamwork and imagination a word like "FLOWERPOTEARTHBREAKER" could be created. The group decides beforehand how many seconds are allowed to think of a letter. No long thinking periods should occur. If the word cannot be continued, it is stopped and a new round is started. In this version verbal communication – apart from naming the letters – is not allowed.

This version can also be played in teams. Which group can make the longest word in a certain time? Discontinued words can also be counted. One point per letter is given. This only applies, however, if the last player is able to spontaneously name the word which should have been created.

Material: A ball of wool.

Move!

Task: The group stands in a circle. One after the other each person moves to the centre, says his or her name and makes some kind of a movement – e.g. snapping their fingers, stamping their foot, turning on the spot ... All the others say the name in chorus and copy the movement. In their thoughts they link the name and the movement and try to remember the combination.

When everyone has introduced themselves with a movement the next round follows, this time with a ball. A makes eye contact with any person in the circle and says "I'm going to throw the ball to Fred – and now move!" The group must now remember the appropriate movement and do it. If it was the right movement, A throws the ball to Fred. If the movement was wrong, it must first be corrected and carried out again together. If nobody can remember it, Fred must help. Then the game continues and Fred seeks a target for his throw: "I'm going to throw the ball to Petra – and now move! This goes on until all have had several turns.

Note: It is of course allowed to ask if a name has been forgotten. It is a good idea to pick those group members to throw the ball to whose names one cannot think of. Through repetition the names are remembered.

Variation 1: As above, but each person is linked not only with one movement, but with two.

Variation 2: As above, but the person whose turn it is to throw shows the movement instead of saying the person's name. The group then calls the name in chorus. Only then does A throw to B.

Variation 3: As above, but the person whose turn it is can choose between starting with the name or the movement – when there are two movements per person, they can even choose between the name and two movements. Then the group has to provide the other movement and the name.

Material: A ball.

Balls, Balls, Balls

Task: The group stands in a circle. A ball is passed around as quickly as possible. More balls are continuously added which must be taken and passed on. The size and material of the balls should vary as much as possible – medicine ball, table tennis ball, water ball, softball, gymnastic ball, balloon, football ...

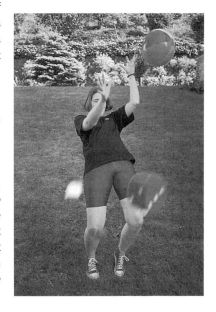

Variation 1:
As above, but the balls are thrown and caught.

Variation 2:
As above, but there is no order. Instead the balls are passed to anyone. It is perfectly all right if the number of balls and the unsystematic passing causes a little chaos – that wakes up the brain! Then, after a short stop, only gradually reintroduce the balls to the game.

Variation 3: As above, but the different types of ball are thrown differently – the medicine ball with both hands from below, the table tennis ball with the left hand, thrown from between the thumb and index finger, the gymnastic ball is thrown with the right hand under the right lower leg etc.

Material: A number of balls of varying sizes and material.

 ### Round as a Ball

Task: The group stands in a circle. The task is to pass a ball around – it can be a table tennis ball, a tennis ball, a water ball, a gymnastic ball, or a billiard ball or similar. It may only be touched with both thumbs, clamped between them and passed on. The next person takes the ball with their thumbs and passes it on in the same way. How many rounds can the group manage without the ball dropping?

The degree of difficulty can be determined by the choice of the ball – its weight, surface, size etc.

Variation 1: As above, but instead of the thumbs only the index fingers, the middle fingers, the ring fingers or the little fingers may be used.

Variation 2: As in 1, but the fingers used are changed in every round – if possible without announcement beforehand – in the first round the thumbs, then the index fingers etc.

Variation 3: As above, but several different balls go round simultaneously.

Variation 4: As above, but two teams are formed. Which team is more skilled and manages the most rounds?

Material: One or more different types of ball.

Coloured Balloons

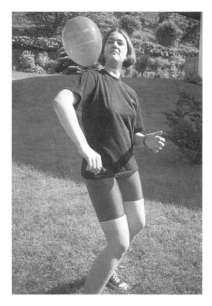

Task: The group stands in a circle. A balloon is kept in the air by hitting it to each other. First the hands are used, then with every contact with the balloon a different part of the body is used, e.g. shoulder, elbow, knee ...

Variation 1:
As above, but with 2, 3, 4, 5 ... balloons; none of them are allowed to touch the ground. In a larger group two teams can be formed. Which team can keep the balloons in the air longest? Which team loses more points (a point is lost every time a balloon touches the ground).

Variation 2: As above, but the formation walks or runs around the room during the game.

Variation 3: Two balloons are used. On one of them a large R is written with a marker pen, on the other an L. The balloon with R may only be touched and hit with the right hand, the one with the L only with the left hand. To recognise them more easily they can be different colours. Would you like a little chaos? Then you can agree that the R balloon can only be hit on the left side and the L balloon only on the right side!

Variation 4: Two, later more different coloured balloons are used. The balloons are thrown, not hit. Using eye contact, the group must agree who throws whom a balloon when, for only one may be thrown at a time. Whoever catches the balloon names a fruit or flower which has the same colour. Thus if someone gets a yellow balloon, and the group has agreed on fruit, banana, sea buckthorn or yellow plum could be the right answer. If flowers have been chosen, someone getting a blue balloon might name forget-me-not, larkspur or iris.

If two or more group members throw their balloon at the same time, both receive minus points. More minus points are given if someone says a wrong word, e.g. daffodils with a red balloon. Who will finish the round with the least points?

Material: Coloured balloons, various colours and marker pens for writing on them.

The Clock Strikes

Task: The group stands in a circle. One after the other each group member throws two large foam dice into the middle. The numbers on the dice are added together. The sum is a time of the day, e.g. a 5 and a 3 equal 8 i.e. 8 o'clock. The player mimes what she or he usually does at this time of day. The group must guess what the activity is. Whoever throws the dice can choose if 8 is 8 a.m. or 8 p.m.

Variation 1:
As above, but with four dice. Then there is no choice of a.m. or p.m. (24 hour clock).

Variation 2:
As above, but small dice are used instead of large foam dice that are visible to all. This way only the person whose turn it is and their neighbour see the time for the pantomime. The group does not have this information. Without knowing the time they have to guess the activity from the movements.

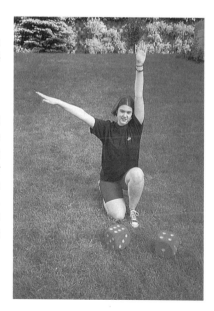

Variation 3: The times of day are determined by the dice as above. All group members form the time as quickly as possible with their arms as it would appear on a clock face. For 12 o'clock both arms point upwards. For 9 o'clock the right arm is held out sideways at shoulder level, the left points up vertically etc. The group must agree from which position the clock is to be seen. It is best if it is visible to the person opposite. How often does the clock show the time completely wrong or is back to front?

Variation 4: As above with two dice. This time the numbers on the dice stand for the months instead of the time, i.e. one for January, two for February ... twelve for December. Each person throws the dice in turn and the whole group must constantly be alert, for all those born in a particular month thrown must move to the centre as quickly as possible.

 ### *Alert Back*

Task: The players form pairs. A and B stand behind each other. A writes a large clear number on B's back with his or her index finger. B tries to feel the number and say it to A. If B guesses wrong the first time, he or she gets a second and third try. One figure numbers should be started with. After some practice, two, three, four and more figure numbers can be felt and remembered. After every figure A taps on B's shoulder as a sign that it is finished. After each message has been felt, A and B exchange roles as transmitter and receiver.

Variation 1: The game can also be used to train the attention span (see page 41). For this the group members must be so well trained that their speed in writing and feeling the numbers is enough to keep to a rate of one, figure per second. Four to six figures are then written. As soon as A has written the last number, B immediately names the number sequence as well as she or he can remember.

Variation 2: As above, but instead of numbers letters are written, later – just as the numbers were extended – words or even short sentences are formed. When training the attention span, letters with no relation to each other are named, if possible without vowels, so that unpronounceable nonsense words are created and no strategies can be used.

Variation 3: The message to be transmitted is not alphanumeric (i.e. neither numbers nor letters). Instead a symbol or a simple picture is drawn.

Variation 4: The message transmitted from A is not named by B. Instead it is answered on the other "alert back" by B: A writes on B's back "1 + 4 x 3" and B answers non-verbally by writing the correct answer "15" on A's back.

Variation 5: When using letters words can be completed. A writes"GYMC", and B adds "LUB". Another possibility is to create a chain of words. A writes "LAND", B writes "SCAPE" (landscape); A continues with "GOAT" (scapegoat) etc.

Note: The game can also be played in a circle. The information is then passed on from one person to the next. Is the message at the end the same as at the beginning?

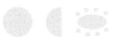

Touch Kim

Task: Various different materials and devices are hidden under a large cloth, such as a bat, ball, double clapper, ... They must be recognised by feeling the top of the cloth with closed eyes (objects that are hard to recognise can be felt under the cloth).

Variation 1:
Teams are formed. Which team recognises all the objects first?

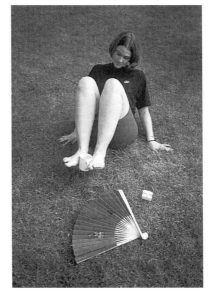

Variation 2: There are two of every object, one under the cloth and one next to it visible to all. The visible objects must be arranged in the same order as those under the cloth.

Variation 3: As in the original version, but with closed eyes the feet are used instead of the hands to feel the cloth. Of course that is only possible if you take your shoes off!

Aura

Task: Pairs stand face to face. A and B stretch their hands in front of them and press the palms of their hands together. They stay in this position for a few seconds. Then A stands still while B takes three steps backwards with closed eyes, then three steps forwards again and tries to find A's hands. Here too the eyes remain closed.

Variation 1:
As above, but the palms of the hands do not touch each other. A and B try to feel the "aura" without physical contact.

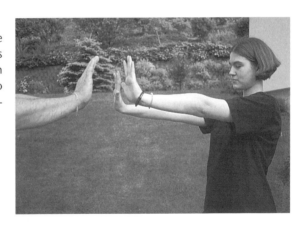

Variation 2: As above, but in addition to walking backwards a complete turn (360°) is carried out. Only then are the hands of the other person sought.

Variation 3: As above, but both A and B close their eyes.

Marionette

Task: Pairs are formed. A lies on a mat on the floor and pretends to be a marionette. B acts as puppeteer and pulls on imaginary strings, thus moving arms, legs or head into various positions, in which the marionette remains briefly.

Material: One mat per pair.

 Mirror Image

Task: The trainer explains a situation in which someone stands in front of a mirror. For example, you get up in the morning and stand opposite your sleepy image before a large wardrobe with mirror doors. In order to wake up, you slowly begin some exercises.

The group members act this situation out, standing in pairs facing each other. A begins with slow flowing movements, for example with an arm. B tries to mirror this in as synchronised a manner as possible. That is why slow movement is necessary. Later other parts of the body are included. How long does a pair take to find out which arm the "mirror" must raise in order to be a real mirror? The faster the movement becomes and the more limbs are involved, the more confusion there is.

Variation 1: The pairs invent their own situations to mirror: Nervousness in the car in a traffic jam when late for an appointment, waiting at a busstop, trying on new clothes in a shop ...

Variation 2: One partner thinks up a situation, the other partner follows it blindly and afterwards has to guess what it was.

Variation 3: As above, but one pair acts out the situation and the other group members guess what it is.

 Sign Language

Task: The group walks or runs around the room. All players are silent. While moving around they try to make eye contact with someone else and in this way form pairs. When all have formed pairs, they interview each other silently. Using only mimicry they must establish who will ask the questions. Both the interviewer and the interviewee are silent and can only communicate with sign language. When each has asked and answered a question, the pairs split up and new pairs are formed. There are no time limits. If someone finds no partner, she or he moves about the room until a new partner is available.

The kind of questions is left up to the participants. What is your occupation? What do you like watching on TV? Which sports do you like best? ...

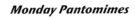

Monday Pantomimes

Task: Two teams are formed. The trainer has prepared a number of cards, on each of which an everyday object is pictured or described with a word, e.g. vacuum cleaner, truck, telephone ... One team member draws a card and uses mime to try and demonstrate the object in such a way that the team can guess it as quickly as possible. When it has been guessed, the next team member has a turn. If the mime uses language to help the team guess, a point is taken off at the end. Every object guessed gains a point. How many objects can be guessed in three minutes? After three minutes it is the turn of the opposing team to try their luck. As a matter of honour the others guess too – but quietly, and without giving hints.

Variation 1: As above, but without a time limit. The teams take turns. Can all the objects be guessed?

Variation 2: As in Variation 1, but for every presentation there are 60 seconds. If an object has not been guessed, the other team carries on.

Variation 3: As above, but instead of just objects proverbs, sayings, first lines of songs etc. must be guessed.

Parcel Post

Task: Two teams are formed which stand in two rows opposite each other. The teams are working at the post office in a special section and in pantomime must pass parcels along which are difficult to transport - without packaging of course. In each team, however, only the "foreman" or "forewoman" knows what each item is. The other team members must guess it.

The trainer has prepared cards on which the objects to be transported are described. The most impossible objects can be posted – a hot cup of tea, a bunch of roses, a handful of rice, a barrel of beer with a hole in it etc. Taking turns, the person at the head of each team draws a card, reads what is to be transported and in pantomime passes this object on. The other team members do not know what they are passing on, but try to guess it as soon as it has reached the end of the chain. After brief consultation amongst themselves they must make a guess. Three guesses are allowed. If they get the answer, the team receives one point and it is the other team's turn

Variation: As above, but instead of a competition between two teams it is played in a circle. Will the group find the answer together?

 ### *Charades*

Task: Depending on the group size, two or more teams are formed. Each team draws a card from the trainer. The word on it must then be presented in pantomime and guessed by the other teams.

The word must be divided into its letters. In the correct order the letters are then individually presented by demonstrating an activity beginning with the respective letter. If for example the word to be demonstrated and guessed is "HER", the three letters are demonstrated one after the other in pantomime. 1st letter = H for holding or hitting; 2nd letter = E for eating or enjoying; 3rd letter = R for riding or rolling.

The other teams watch the group's presentations and try to guess the word. If it is not guessed, the trainer can help with a few hints.

Variation 1: As above, but the letters of the word are not presented in the correct order. Instead they are mixed up in a jumble. The guessing teams must therefore not only work out the letters but also put them in the right order.

Variation 2: Instead of words, whole sentences or sayings are pantomimed word for word. In doing so, the individual pantomime presentations must of course correspond to the real meaning of the word in each case.

Recognise the Ball

Task: The group close their eyes. One after another the trainer drops different types of balls on the ground – a table tennis ball, a basketball, a medicine ball ... Everyone tries to recognise the type of ball from the sound it makes. The exercise is easier if the balls are all shown to the group beforehand.

Variation: The balls must be recognised by their shape and texture through feeling instead of by their sound. For this either everyone must close their eyes or the balls must be hidden in a blanket or cardboard box.

Material: Various types of balls, if necessary a cardboard box or sack to hide them in.

Noise Orchestra

Task: The group sits – in the formation of an orchestra – looking towards the trainer, who initially acts as a conductor. Various symbols are written as "notes" on a poster (see example in Appendix, page 129) that functions as "sheet music". Each symbol represents a particular movement or a noise: Drum for slapping the thighs, trumpet for stamping the right foot, guitar for snapping the fingers etc. If using a blackboard more simple symbols such as or can of course be used.

A group member sets the tone, and the orchestra responds: If the conductor points at the drum, all slap their thighs, if he points at the trumpet they all stamp loudly with their right foot etc. The noise range can be as comprehensive as the group wishes, including clapping hands or slapping the thighs, stamping with the left or right foot, snapping the fingers, clicking the tongue, whistling etc.

Variation: As above, but materials for creating noises are also used.

Blooming Coloured Glory

Task: The group forms a circle. All players choose a flower for themselves. One after another the plants and their colours are named: e.g yellow daffodil, blue larkspur, white marguerites etc. If possible, only well known plants should be chosen and in smaller groups none should be included twice or more. It is advantageous if many different coloured blooms are chosen. Plenty of time should be allowed for presenting the flowers and their colours so that all pieces of information can be taken in and memorised step by step. When the colours are named, it is useful to point at the appropriate colour in the room, e.g. for red to go up to a person in a red T-shirt, point to it and say "I am a red poppy".

The trainer calls out any colour and the appropriate people walk past each other and swap places. For yellow this might be e.g. buttercups, daffodils, cowslips and forsythias. For blue it could be violets, larkspurs and irises. If anyone misses their move, they take the trainer's place and call out the next colours.

Variation 1: As above, but there are no verbal commands. Instead coloured balloons, boards, cloths or similar are held up and all must quickly respond to this visual information.

Variation 2: As above, but instead of naming colours the trainer calls out a player's name. If for example Mary is called out, who has presented herself as a white chrysanthemum, then she must change places with any other flower with the same colour. She has a choice of Peter, the white lilac and Jill, the white rhododendron. If she goes up to a person whose petals are not white, she takes over the trainer's position and calls out the next person's name.

Variation 3: As in Variation 2, but the place changing in every round is continued until all flowers with a particular colour have found a new place.

Variation 4: As in Variation 2, but when Mary, the white chrysanthemum, is called out, she does not move. Instead everyone else must remember what colour she chose and all with the same colour - in this case white – must change places.

Variation 5: As above, but instead of flowers e.g. fruits are chosen – yellow bananas, red cherries, green kiwifruit, blue plums etc.

Note: Depending on the group, it may be advisable for the trainer to allot the plants, fruits etc. by letting the players draw cards. This ensures that all colours are included and that they are relatively evenly spread.

Zip Zap

Task: The group stands in a circle. The idea is to get to know each other better. Each group member asks their neighbours left and right a personal question which must be briefly answered, e.g. about their hobbies, taste in music, favourite pets, star sign ... and memorises this information. The trainer stands in the middle of the circle. She or he goes up to a group member, who must react as quickly as possible and loudly call out the required information. If the trainer says "Zip", the person addressed must say something about the person to their left, if the trainer says "Zap", they must say something about the person on their right. The trainer should ensure rapid change. No one is allowed to think too long, for anyone who needs a lot of time must change places with the trainer.

The game really gets moving when the trainer calls out "Zip Zap". When they hear this command, the players must run amongst themselves and exchange places. Then of course, they first have to get information about their new neighbours.

Variation 1: As above, but two pieces of information are asked of each person instead of just one. In this case it must first be agreed what kind of information is to be asked, e.g. info 1 = shoe size, info 2 = birthday or similar. The trainer's commands are then e.g. "Zip 1", "Zip 2", "Zap 1" and "Zap 2". That makes it much more difficult to answer quickly!

Variation 2: As above, but instead of verbal information, movement information is given and repeated. When asked about the date of birth for example the answer could be given by writing it in the air with one's finger or the question about one's hobby could be replied to with a brief pantomime.

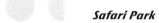

Safari Park

Task: The trainer tells a brief story about a visit to the zoo or a trip to an exotic country which is home to many animals. A safari park is visited. The group acts out the situation together. All stand in a circle. First the trainer stands in the middle, later other group members take turns. The task is to represent certain animals or plants when an appropriate command is given. In each case three people are required to react as quickly as possible to jointly carry out the proper movements. The trainer points at a person in the circle and calls out e.g. "lion", "palm tree" or "elephant". The person pointed to carries out the main movement, those on his or her left and right are the complementing figures.

- The main palm tree raises both arms, the complementing palm trees each raise the arm closest to the main palm tree. All three sway in the wind together.
- The main elephant holds his nose with one hand and puts his other arm through this one as a trunk. Complementing elephants use their arms to indicate large ears.
- The main lion jumps through an imaginary ring created by the complementing lions. Complementing lions use their arms to create a ring for the main lion to jump through.
- ... Further figures can be invented by the group.

I Say Shoulder

Task: The group stands in such a way that all can easily see the trainer. A circle is good, but standing in a row is also possible.

The players must all obey "orders" in such a way that they always do what the trainer says, but not what she or he does. If for example the trainer says "shoulder" and actually touches her or his shoulder, so does everybody else. If, however, she or he says "shoulder" but touches her or his hip for example, all group members should touch their shoulders (and not their hips!!!).

All movements can be one-sided or double sided, i.e. carried out with the left or the right hand or foot or with both extremities at the same time. If a decision on right or left is required the exercise is more difficult than with both simultaneously.

The more quickly the directions are given, the more difficult – and more fun – the game is.

Mobile groups can play moving around, less mobile groups can do it standing still or if necessary in a sitting position. Through the choice of the parts of the body or the movements, the trainer can determine the amount of effort required and adjust this to match the group.

Variation 1: The task is reversed, i.e. everyone must do what is shown and not what is said.

Variation 2: As above, but instead of touching parts of the body movements are carried out. The trainer says e.g. "I say: go", but remains standing or "I say: lift your right arm", "I say: sit", "I say: clap" etc. and combines these commands with the appropriate or another movement. The others must quickly decide in each case which movement they should actually carry out.

The Traffic Lights Are Out Of Order

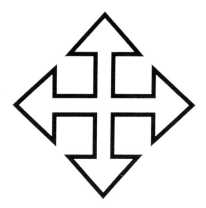

Task: The trainer tells the group a story about how – while going into town – one day the traffic lights were out of order. There was traffic chaos, so she or he finally directed the traffic.

The group acts out the situation together. The trainer points to the appropriate arrow and all stretch their arms in the required direction as quickly as possible: up, down, right and left.

Fig. 11 (created by Bettina M. Jasper using Cliparts from Corel Draw, Corel Corporation, Canada)

Note: The movement is accompanied by language, with each direction "up", "down", "right" or "left" being spoken, in order to increase the supply of blood to the brain (see motoric homunculus, page 22).

Variation 1: As above, but all do exactly the opposite of what is pointed to - the arms go up when down has been pointed to etc.; at the same time the opposite is also spoken.

Variation 2: As above, but what is shown is spoken while the arms move in the opposite direction.

Variation 3: The arrow tips are coloured and the direction is not shown but called out, e.g. "red", "green" etc. or indicated by holding up coloured boards or cloths etc. Of course it can be agreed that "red" always means "green" and "yellow" always means "blue" etc. All clear?

Material: Poster with four different coloured arrows (could be made with foil or similar).

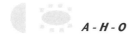 **A - H - O**

Task: The group stands in a circle. The letters A, H and O are quickly called out in sequence again and again. The order in which the group members call out the letters is determined by the gestures. The group decides who starts.

For the three letters A, H and O gestures are agreed on. Calling out the letter and carrying out the appropriate movement should be done as quickly as possible.
    A = optionally placing the back of one's left or right hand under one's chin. The fingertips thus point to the neighbour to the right or left, depending on which hand is used. According to the direction indicated here, the game continues. The player pointed to continues by calling out H.
H = like A, i.e. optionally placing the left or right hand under one's chin.

The person now pointed to carries on with O. O means: stretch out an arm and point to anyone in the circle, with whom the game begins at A again.

This way the three letters are named again and again in fast sequence. The order within the circle changes constantly as it is left up to every player to determine the direction of the game.

Variation 1: A and H can be called out and accompanied by gestures as often as desired. Whoever's turn it is decides when another part of the circle is included by using the signal O.

Variation 2: The letters are replaced by numbers. The players count. 1 begins with his or her hand under the chin, 2 carries on in any direction with the same movement. 3 points to someone else in the circle. 4 and 5 carry on with a hand under their chin, at 6 someone in the circle must be pointed to again. Thus the group keeps counting, and at every number divisible by 3 a finger is pointed.

Variation 3: As above, but numbers can be called out in any order. All numbers divisible by 3 are accompanied by pointing a finger, all others by placing a hand under the chin.

8 The Brain Fitness Circuit – Thinking and Exercise at 1 + 10 Stations

8.1 The Idea and the Combinations

The Brain Fitness Circuit is a form of station training in which thinking and exercise are combined. In contrast to other training and game examples in this book, all – or at least several – of the stations are intended to be used in a single training session or event. Nevertheless, it is of course possible to pick out individual stations and include them in a "normal" training session.

The idea of the Brain Fitness Circuit is to compactly take up the topic of thinking and exercise and bring it to the attention of the participants. Station training is a useful way for a group or club to first approach the topic. In direct conjunction with or shortly after or before the Circuit, related talks and courses can be offered such as:
• a lecture about mental challenges in daily life and special training options;
• a lecture about links between mental and physical fitness;
• a lecture about links between mental and physical fitness with nutrition;
• a course on training brain performance;
• a group meeting to train mental fitness;
• ...

And in any case, after such an introduction, every training session should include at least one brief activity which trains the brain. An appropriate comment from the trainer each time to encourage people to think about the necessity of mental training and to create ongoing motivation is also necessary.
    The Brain Fitness Circuit can also be simply a variation of the regular training session.

The description of the various stations has deliberately been kept vague with as few concrete details as possible. This is to keep things flexible and not dependent on particular devices, rooms or materials. This deliberately contrived flexibility means that in spite of certain directions, trainers have creative leeway and in fact their creativity is called for.

Station training is not meant to be considered a test, i.e. the combinations can be changed around. It can and should also be an inspiration to group and trainer to develop their own ideas for other stations and so one day to create a completely new Brain Fitness Circuit.

Thus for example the "Buttonhole" of Station 3 can be replaced without a problem by "Pearl Necklace" , in which as many wooden beads as possible must be threaded together as quickly as possible, or by "Bow Tying", where prepared ribbons and strings must be bound into bows. All stations can be varied in a similar way.

Intentionally, no points are awarded because it is not a test and the results cannot be compared anyway. The main thing is having fun. Nevertheless, everyone will make an effort and do their best.

The stations are done in pairs, whereby both partners are always active, sometimes simultaneously and together, sometimes alternating with different tasks. If there are more than 20 people in a group, the number of stations can be increased.

Every player needs a games list and a pen. Either two pens can be placed at each station or (more reliable!) the players take their pens from station to station.

The games lists are photocopied and a copy given to each person. An example is shown in the Appendix on page 130.

In addition, worksheets are required at various stations. There must also be at least one copy per person of these.

It helps if the group has already been made aware on earlier occasions of the kinds of exercises used for mental training so that everyone knows what to do e.g. with an alphabet square or an exercise "Crossing out number patterns". Questions during the Circuit disturb the flow and should be avoided. At the latest when describing the Brain Fitness Circuit before beginning with it, the exercises for mental training should be explained in detail and demonstrated with the help of examples in order to avoid misunderstandings as far as possible.

All activities begin together at Station 1. Then the pairs, who have been drawn or designated, spread themselves around the other ten stations. The trainer gives the signals for changing stations or partners. The length of the time units can be decided under consideration of factors such as the fitness of the group, the space available, the equipment used etc. As a rule it should be between two and three minutes per task, i.e. between five and seven minutes per station, including partner change. The beginning and end of each time unit can be signalled by calling it out or by an agreed acoustic signal such as a whistle, beating a drum etc. For changing pairs from station to station music has proven to be suitable.

During each time unit the pairs carry out the tasks of their particular station. When the stop signal is given, they stop what they are doing, no matter how far they have got with it. There is no requirement of perfection in the Brain Fitness Circuit! Everyone needs a different amount of time for the various tasks and so there will be differences in how far each person gets with them. This applies to both the physical and the mental tasks.

For example, at Station 3 some will manage to complete one column of number patterns in their worksheet, others will get the second or even third column done. In the same way, there is bound to be a difference in the number of direction changes in the balancing act at Station 10. The same applies to all stations. At Station 4 not everyone will work out the answer – and thus the result of the bucket run. But the training of the brain happens regardless of the result! The effect is achieved by thinking, not by finding the answer.

The tasks have intentionally been selected in such a way and with such an amount to do that they cannot always be completed.

It is important that the games lists and worksheets can be taken home afterwards. In this way everyone has an opportunity to go through the tasks again afterwards and finish any uncompleted exercises. In addition, it can encourage people to carry on with mental training independent of the sports session and to acquire appropriate material themselves. Sources for such materials can be found in the address section on page 139. Anyone who has had experience with alphabet squares in everyday life, such as in magazines, will be more at ease with this kind of task than someone doing it for the first time. The same goes for all other types of tasks.

With the help of the games list, tasks involving movement can be trained at home. Buttons for sorting or doing up can be found in practically every household. Lines for balancing on can be found on any street paving or be drawn or made by placing a rope on a lawn.

The Brain Fitness Circuit should thus not be considered just a one-off event to be forgotten about afterwards, but should encourage regular training during the day. Talking about it in the group environment is an important step in this direction. The trainer should always take the initiative if it does not come from the group itself.

8.2 The Stations

Station 1 - Picture Board

Material: Large poster with 20 picture squares which also each contain a number. (Example: see Appendix, page 131) To ensure easier recognition when the group is somewhat larger, the pictures can be enlarged on a photocopier and hung on the wall as 20 individual sheets.

Organisational Form: Complete group at once, all at the Start Station.

Task: Everyone gets in a position from where they can see the pictures well. When the start signal is given, they begin to walk or run on the spot. Simultaneously, the pictures are looked at intensely and memorised. The idea is to memorise as many as possible, including the number linked to each picture. Two time units are allowed for this task.

Station 2 - Peggy Sue

Material: Five clothes pegs; one worksheet "Alphabet Squares" per person (Example: see Appendix, page 132).

Organisational Form: Two people, A and B, together.

Tasks: 1. The partners peg themselves together with the clothes pegs and try to move together as quickly as possible without losing the pegs.

2. A and B each take a worksheet with an alphabet square. In this words are hidden, as many of which as possible must be found and circled. The sheets should be taken along when finished, not left lying for the next team with found words marked!

Station 3 - Buttonhole

Material: Old pillowcases and continental quilt covers, clothes and similar with many buttons and buttonholes; one worksheet "Crossing out number patterns" per person (Example: see Appendix, page 133).

Organisational Form: A and B simultaneously.

Tasks: 1. A and B each take a pillow case or continental quilt cover or similar and quickly button up as many buttons as possible one after the other. When you are finished undo all the buttons for the next pair!
2. A and B each take a worksheet and rapidly work through the number columns from top to bottom, crossing out the number patterns as shown in the example (cf. training example on page 40 and worksheet on page 133)

Station 4 - Bucket Run

Material: Seven plastic buckets or road markers; seven selected letter cards, foam or wooden letters which together form a word, e.g. the letters LANOTEG = GOALNET (cf.: Exercise "Scrambled letters: sports" in the Appendix, page 134).

Organisational Form: A and B simultaneously.

Tasks: 1. Independently of each other and in a different order, A and B run by the seven buckets or road markers spread around the room. At each one they lift it to briefly see which letter is under it and then put it back down. The seven letters must be memorised for the second task at this station.
2. A and B use the time in this round to write the seven letters they have gathered on their games list and if possible to put them in an order that makes a proper word.

Station 5 - Parts of a Whole

Material: A pillowcase or cottton bag containing a number of empty ballpoint pens – i.e. without the ink refills; a simple puzzle, nine parts, possibly also a cut up postcard or calendar page.

Organisational Form: A and B alternate.

Tasks: 1. A "blindly" screws together as many ballpoint pens as possible inside the pillowcase or cotton bag. When finished, take them apart again for the next player!
2. At the same time B puts the puzzle parts together. When finished, take them apart for the next player!

Station 6 - Ball Test

Material: A ball (gymnastics ball, softball etc.), the station should be set up near a wall; a sheet with a text that has mistakes in it (Example: see Appendix, page 135).

Organisational Form: A and B alternate.

Tasks: 1. During the whole time unit A keeps throwing the ball at the wall and catching it. Various ways of throwing can be tried out - with two hands, with one hand, overarm, underarm, forwards, backwards over the head, under a leg etc.
2. B reads a text. The text contains many mistakes. In almost every word letters have been replaced by strange characters. That makes it harder to read:
Wo➡ld it n③t be m⟳ch e⑦si◀r to re➡d this s▲nte➡ce if a➴ the le♣ters we❺e co⟳ple❷e?

Station 7 - Feeling Box

Material: A cardboard box with holes on two sides for reaching through and about 10 objects (e.g. button, tennis ball, eraser, cork, teaspoon, sandpaper, padlock ...); a "picture board" poster from Station 1 placed so that it cannot be seen.

Organisational Form: A and B alternate.

Tasks: 1. A reaches through the two holes in the cardboard box and feels the objects inside, memorises them until the end of the exercise and then writes them down on his or her games list.

2. When the start signal is given, B turns over the poster with the picture board and looks at it again intensely, adding up the numbers in the 20 squares and writing the result on the games list.

Station 8 - Noticeboard

Material: A large sheet of newspaper per person.

Organisational Form: A and B simultaneously.

Tasks: 1. A and B each unfold a large sheet of newspaper and first hold them against their chests. Then they start moving and cross the room so quickly that the sheet of newspaper does not fall down.

2. In any article – if A and B have the same page they should agree beforehand on the same text – each one crosses out all the capital "A"s and small "a"s.

Station 9 - Buttoneyes

Material: A big box with many different buttons; a poster with seven spaces marked on a "chessboard" (Example: see Appendix, page 136).

Organisational Form: A and B together.

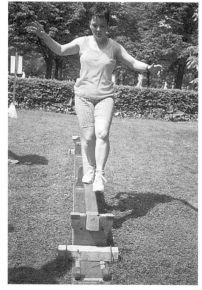

Tasks: 1. The box of buttons is tipped out. Together A and B sort the buttons into pairs or threes. When finished, put all the buttons back in the box for the next pair!

2. A poster with a "chessboard" pattern, i.e. marked spaces in a pattern of 25 squares, lies covered. When the start signal is heard, the poster is uncovered. Together A and B briefly look at it for about ten seconds, then turn it back over. Immediately afterwards and independently of each other, A and B try to mark on the pattern in their games list the same spaces they saw on the poster.

Station 10 - Balancing Act

Material: A bench – normal or turned upside down – or a sideline, if necessary a line taped on the floor or a rope laid out on the grass ...; covered up paper with a topic written on it, about which words/groups of words containing varying amounts of syllables must be found (Example: see Appendix, page 137). The topic should be a situation, e.g. "In the gym".

Organisational Form: A and B alternate.

Tasks: 1. A balances nonstop along the bench, or another route that has been decided on, for the duration of this time unit, i.e. often changing direction, if possible without getting off the bench or line.

2. When the start signal is heard, B uncovers the paper with the topic and reads it. Then he or she has to think of words/groups of words about the topic, e.g. "In the gym", with one syllable, with two syllables etc. up to five syllables, and write them in the games list: 1 = ball, 2 = gym mat, 3 = wooden horse, 4 = basketball hoop, 5 = playing area.

Station 11 - Rope Walking

Material: Two ropes.

Organisational Form: A and B simultaneously.

Tasks: 1. For the duration of the time unit A and B run with the rope on the spot or around the room, without stopping if possible. Of course skipping is allowed. For older participants, however, the version of running with the rope is preferable. The number of times the rope is stepped over should be counted.

2. Independently of each other A and B enter in their games list – if possible in the correct space – which pictures from Station 1 they can still remember. The objects can be drawn or written as a word. Can anyone also put the numbers in the right places?

9 Crack the N(o)ut! – Moving Card Games

Under the title "N(o)usknacker" ("N(o)utcracker") (Source: Denk-Werkstatt, Address see page 139) two card games centre on mind and memory. They were developed by Hanjette Mosmann, Bernd Fischer and Bernhard Dickreiter, the training team of the Memory Clinic Nordrach, on the basis of the latest scientific research and promote general mental performance.

Nousknacker 1 and 2 are games with unlimited possibilities and variations. Originally developed exclusively for mental training as a card game at a table, in a slightly varied form they can be put in to motion in the true sense of the word. The moving versions of Nousknacker show how mental and physical training can be combined.

For the moving Nousknacker versions it can be helpful, but is not necessary, to have the card games available. When playing in a hall, in larger rooms or outside, large cards are needed. These one must make oneself, either by enlarging the original cards on a photocopier and sticking the copies to cardboard, or by drawing similar cards on cardboard using the same characters.

Available original cards are useful for the trainer to have as a model for making the materials for the moving Nousknacker versions, and in order for him or her – at a table – to get familiar with the idea of the games, the effects and the possibilities for variation.

For group members the original cards serve to improve their personal mental performance. Anyone who regularly trains the basic functions of the brain in this way can call on more mental fitness and thus achieve greater personal success.

9.1 Card Games as Basis for Deliberate Training

The original version of the card games for purely training mental performance form the basis for the variations in motion. With them the basic functions of the brain can be trained in accordance with the explanations on page 39 ff.

In the title there is only a number which differentiates Nousknacker 1 and Nousknacker 2 from each other. There are, however, major differences in the idea and the conditions of the games.

First what they have in common: "Nous" comes from Greek and means mind, reason. And this really gets trained. Nevertheless, the games work independently of knowledge and education. Nobody needs to be afraid of making a fool of themselves in front of a group. Both Nousknacker versions are card games. They can be played alone, in pairs or in groups. In each case there is a basic version and variations of it which are described in an accompanying booklet. With a little imagination and creativity, players can discover numerous other forms of the game.

Through deliberate use of numbers, letters, symbols and pictures in Nousknacker 1 and 2 both halves of the brain are always activated. The card games were developed by the team at the Memory Clinic in Nordrach with their Superintendent Prof. Dr. med. Bernd Fischer who established his reputation in particular as one of the founding fathers of Integrated Brain Performance Training (German: Integratives Hirnleistungstraining or IHT®) or Mental Activating Training (MAT).

In spite of all parallels each game has its own attractiveness and its own game idea.

Nousknacker 1

64 playing cards with what at first seems a rather strange appearance are the material. On every card there are five or six figures in constantly varying combinations – numbers, letters and symbols. In comparing the figures on a card on the game pile with one of the basic cards, the main thing is concentration and fast processing of information. Figures should be recognised quickly and the cards placed on a plus and a minus pile.

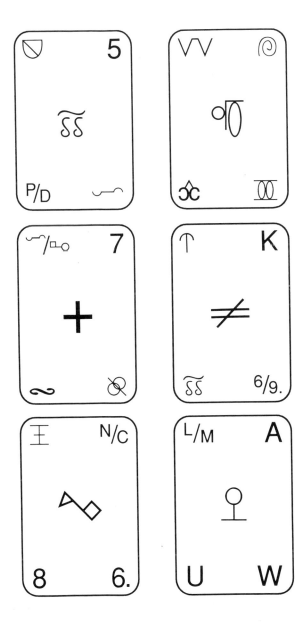

Fig. 12 (with kind permission of Wissiomed GmbH, Prof. Dr. B. Fischer)

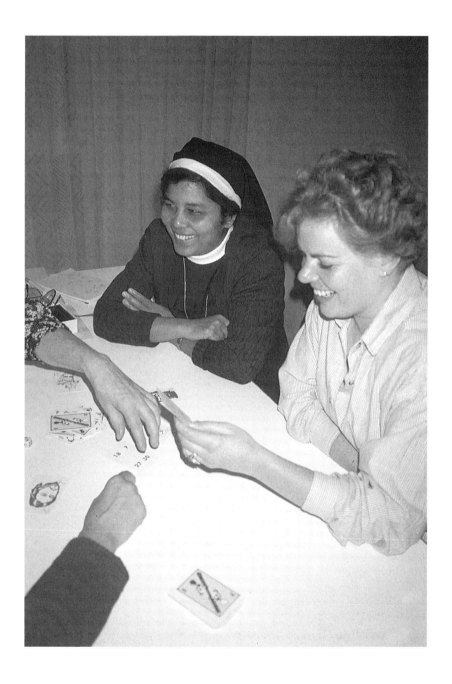

The player's memory is challenged when the basic card(s) – with a little practice two can be used – are turned over after consciously remembering all of the figures on them. Will the cards from the deck still land correctly on the plus and minus pile?

In another variation the short term retention of information is the object of the game. The player looks at the figures on a playing card for a few seconds, turns it over and must then immediately remember what was on the card. Will she or he be able to recollect all the numbers, letters and symbols, and if possible write them down in the correct order and position as on the card?

These and many other versions can be played primarily alone or in pairs. There are, however, versions for three or four persons. A whole range of new combinations makes the game seem different each time, requires even after much repetition – a great deal of attention and develops the powers of concentration.

The short game duration of five to ten minutes per round makes it possible to quickly liven oneself up mentally any time and anywhere.

All in all, it is a fascinating game that can be played anywhere and quickly get you mentally fit. And ... it is a game for which I need not spend time looking for other enthusiasts but can play on my own any time!

Nousknacker 2

For Nousknacker 2, 64 cards are also required and additionally a dice. This is mainly a group game, but can be played alone. More emphasis is placed on having fun than on the – nevertheless present – training value. In the first minutes of the game already there is usually laughter and enjoyment in the group.

In the basic version everything revolves around six easily remembered cards with faces: a fat man with a cigar, a woman with curly hair etc. These cards are laid out in any order in a circle on the table. In the top left corner of each face card there is a picture of a dice, each displaying a different number – the One belongs to the woman with the headscarf, the Two to the Marilyn Monroe imitation etc. There are cards with numbers, letters, syllables, words, symbols and pictures. In the first round, six of these cards, one of

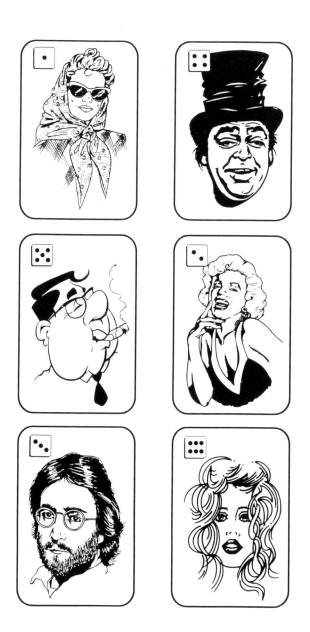

Fig. 13 (With kind permission of Wissiomed GmbH, Prof. Dr. B. Fischer)

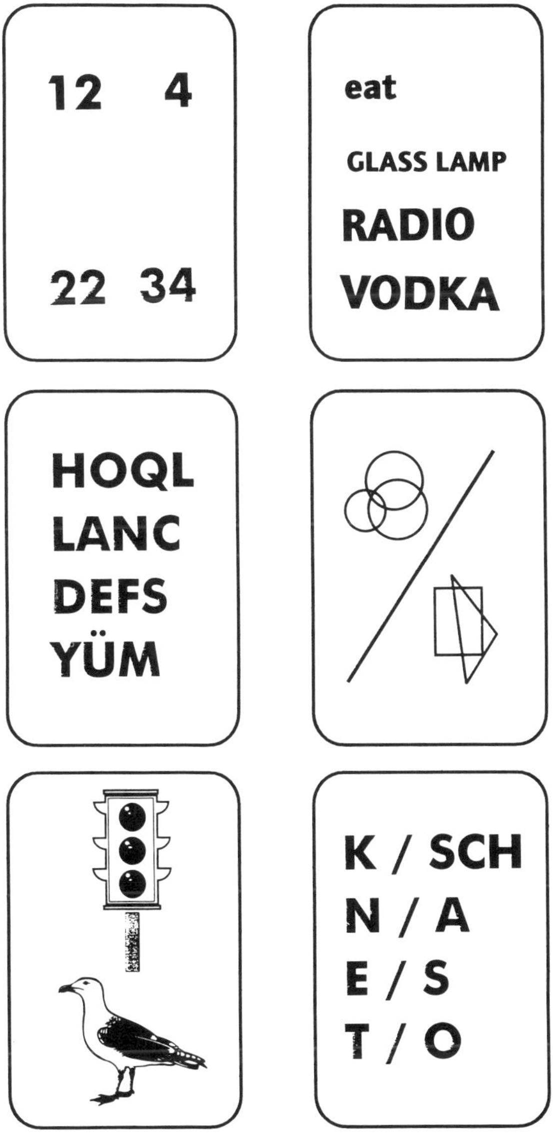

12 4 **22 34**	eat **GLASS LAMP** **RADIO** **VODKA**
HOQL **LANC** **DEFS** **YÜM**	
	K / SCH **N / A** **E / S** **T / O**

Fig. 14 (With kind permission of Wissiomed GmbH, Prof. Dr. B. Fischer)

each type, are placed next to the face cards. After a brief memorising phase each playing card is pushed underneath the appropriate face card thus making it no longer visible. Now the actual game starts. The remaining playing cards are mixed and evenly divided among the players. Now the dice is used. One after another each player must remember which card is hidden under the face card with the dice number they have thrown. Were there pictures under the man with the cigar or were there words after all, ... no, perhaps there were syllables? When the secret is finally revealed, the playing card is taken out from under the face card and replaced by another playing card from the pile of the person who threw the dice. If the person whose turn it was remembered correctly, he or she gets the card and earns points. If he or she got something wrong, the card is removed from the game. When all the piles are finished, the results are evaluated. Who has scored the most points?

The scoring provides for a number of variations. Correct cards can be counted if players have remembered whether words, syllables, numbers ... were involved. This becomes more difficult when an experienced group decides that at least one concrete picture, letter or similar must be named and so on.

The constantly changing game situation requires great attentiveness of all participants. It is usually most fun when someone has again made a mistake.

The accompanying brochure describes further versions which can also be played alone or in pairs. As with Nousknacker 1, here too all basic brain functions can be specifically trained.

Those who prefer to play alone and be independent of whether or not others want to play and who place more value on the training aspect than "just having fun" should choose Nousknacker 1.

Those who mainly want to have fun with occasional games with family, friends and acquaintances and at the same time enjoy a positive effect on their mental performance do well to choose Nousknacker 2.

9.2 The Cards and how They Are Made

For the moving forms of Nousknacker 1 and 2 original playing cards are usually used. For some versions simpler forms or enlargements are needed. These have to be home-made on the basis of the original cards.

If using original cards by hanging them up at various positions, they should be put in plastic sleeves in order to protect them and make them easily visible. The same is recommended when individual characters of the Nousknacker 1 cards are drawn on DIN A4 paper or cardboard.

If enlarged original cards are needed – e.g. the face cards of Nousknacker 2 –, it is possible to enlarge them on a photocopier. In this case it is advisable to use standard sizes: DIN A4 or DIN A5. To make them easier to use they should be stuck onto cardboard. If they are to be used often and need to last longer, they should also be covered with self-adhesive bookbinding film.

Even better – and not necessarily more expensive – is laminating. In this process, which is offered by most copy shops, the paper is sealed in foil and is thus not only stronger but also washable. Anyone using the cards very often or outside should definitely decide on this method.

Those who are not perfectionists or just want to try out the games in their own groups can write or draw the necessary characters on cardboard with a paintbrush or bold marker pen. The same applies when there are no original cards available. Then in addition creativity is required, for symbols must be invented and then combined with letters and numbers.

9.3 Moving Nousknacker

In the following examples, it is not just a matter of fast running and general physical fitness, nor is high mental performance alone the key. Finding the right individual combination of both aspects is the secret of success here.

Game Versions Based on Nousknacker 1

Running after Characters

Task: Before the session, the trainer hangs up about 20 posts around the room or – if outside – on tree trunks etc. Each post consists of a sheet of paper or a card with a character on it. This can be a letter, a number or a symbol. The posts are fastened in such a way that the characters are hidden, i.e. cannot be seen from a distance already, but must be briefly lifted on arriving at the post in order to be seen.

The group is given a certain amount of time, e.g. three to five minutes, depending on the size of the room or the area where the posts are hung. In the available time every player tries to run around as many characters as possible and remember them. When the finishing signal is given all meet at a certain point. There the trainer briefly distracts the group, e.g. with a sum to be done in one's head.

Only then is the group divided among previously laid out sheets and pens, and each writes or draws all of the characters he or she can remember. For this phase also a certain length of time is allocated, e.g. 60 seconds. For every correct character a point is awarded, for every wrong one a point is subtracted.

It is therefore of little use if someone runs really fast and manages to run around all the posts in the available time if these cannot all be remembered after the distraction phase. Only with a certain amount of practice can a person find the right measure for their own performance, the right combination of using mental and physical fitness. Also, you need good planning and good observation of the other players so that not all turn up at the same post at the same time and cause a tussle over who gets to see the character first.

Variation 1: As above, but only numbers are used. In this case the numbers may be double digits.

Variation 2: As above, but only symbols are used. Then, however, the game should begin with less posts.

Variation 3: As above, but the game is played in teams which are not allowed to verbally communicate during the running phase. The individual scores are added to make team results. Which team will score highest?

Variation 4: As in Variation 3, but in pairs instead of teams.

Variation 5: As above, but the characters need not be actively written down or drawn. Instead the trainer hands out prepared sheets on which many more than the 20 characters actually displayed are to be found. In multiple choice fashion the players mark the characters they remember. Right and wrong answers are scored just as in the first version.

Variation 6: As above, but certain letters, which can be formed into a word, are included amongst the c. 20 characters. For example, the letters E, O, R, M could be hung up together with other characters. Whoever writes one of the two possible words "ROME" or "MORE" on their sheet gets five extra points, if they get both words, they receive ten extra points.

Variation 7: As above, but there are extra points for those who can add up all the numbers which were hung up. For example, if in addition to other characters the numbers 7, 12, 3, 22 and 53 were included and someone writes down the total of 97, they receive five valuable extra points. But be careful: Don't concentrate so hard on the numbers that you forget the other characters!

Variation 8: As above, but instead of 20 posts only ten are distributed. These, however, each include two characters. In the evaluation there is – as in the original version – an additional point for each correct character, but also a point for each correct combination of characters.

Variation 9: As above, but for the last part of the game, recalling the characters covered, instead of empty pages sketches of the room or area with the posts are distributed. The players try not only to remember as many characters as possible, but receive an extra point for every character for which they can remember the right location.

Nousknacker Relay

Task: Teams of three or four stand lined up. At the start signal the first person in each team runs to a point roughly ten metres away, which can be marked e.g. with a crate or a tyre. At this point there is a deck of Nousknacker 1 cards. The first player picks up the top card and looks at it – approximately one second per character on the card – then runs back to their team with the card, which must then be kept covered and not looked at again. The player puts the card aside and, as quickly as possible, writes from memory the characters – numbers, letters and symbols – on a piece of paper which has been prepared beforehand. As soon as the first player has put down the pen, the second person can start running. For each card a new piece of paper is used. When the first team has finished all its cards the game is ended and the results are evaluated.

For the evaluation a card is placed next to the appropriate sheet of paper. For each recognisably written character a point is awarded, for each wrong character a point is subtracted. Which team has written down the most characters correctly?

Variation: As above, but the characters must be written down in exactly the same position as on the card. Points are only given for characters in the correct position.

Note: For this game it is best to use the original Nousknacker 1 cards. It also helps if the cards that only contain symbols, i.e. no letter or numbers, are removed beforehand and not used. Because of the different combinations of characters the cards differ in difficulty. Therefore not only the fitness of the teams but also partially chance and luck determine the outcome.

Before they are divided amongst the teams the cards should be shuffled for everyone to see. Depending on the number of participants, one set of cards is usually enough, for larger groups use two. Approximately three cards per player are enough.

8 x 6

Task: The trainer spreads as many Nousknacker 1 cards around the room or outside as there are people playing. The cards lie or are hung up so that they cannot be seen and practically form a parcours. They should follow an easily recognisable imaginary line. To make it easier to find the cards, numbered street markers can be placed over them (under the markers the cards can be placed face up).

Each player has a photocopied sheet of paper with eight empty playing card spaces (see example in Appendix, page 140) on a hard background and a pen. At each card one person is positioned. All group members must look at each of eight cards for a few seconds, cover up the card and immediately write the characters seen on it in one of the spaces on their sheet. They have to run a short distance between each card.

The trainer is responsible for timing and giving the stop and go signals. During the running phases music is played. When the music stops, each player goes to the next station. On the agreed signal, they turn over the card and look at it for about six or seven seconds. After the signal for covering up the cards, the players have a few seconds to write the character on their sheets. Then the music signals that it is time to run to the next position. This rhythm continues until eight card positions have been covered. At the end, everyone compares their sheet with the cards at the various positions. For every correct character a point is awarded, with an additional point for every correct position, and minus points for incorrect characters.

Laying the Cards "Blind"

Task: At twelve positions around the room, randomly chosen characters from the Nousknacker 1 cards are placed for all to see. The group runs or quickly walks around the room to music for five to ten minutes.

Each player consciously passes the various positions several times and memorises the characters. When the music stops, pairs are formed, each sharing a deck of Nousknacker 1 cards, i.e. 32 cards each. As quickly as possible, they each "blindly" sort their cards into plus and minus cards, i.e. without looking around the room.

The twelve characters that have been memorised form the basis – or have some been forgotten already? Cards containing at least one of the twelve characters are plus cards; minus cards are those which display none of the characters seen in the room. After quickly sorting, each player slowly goes through their minus pile to check it, consciously comparing the cards with the characters around the room to see how many cards or characters have been missed out.

Material: One Nousknacker 1 card deck per two players.

Game Versions Based on Nousknacker 2

Who's Who?

Task: Small groups of five or six people form circles. Within each circle the six enlarged face cards from Nousknacker 2 (see illustration on page 108/109) are randomly laid out on the ground, also in a circle. First the group agrees on names for the card faces. In this version, it is advisable not to choose the names of prominent people who look similar to those on the cards, but rather to choose other names. When all of the faces have been clearly "identified", the game can begin. Each person throws a dice. The person who has thrown names the name of the appropriate face, e.g. for four the name of the man in the top hat. If the name is confused or cannot be remembered at all, the person receives a punishment. The group decides before the game what that will be, e.g. crawl around the circle on hands and knees, run around the circle balancing something etc. If the correct name is named, the game continues and the next person throws the dice.

Usually, after just a few rounds everyone knows all the names and the degree of difficulty has to be increased in order to bring more movement into the game through "punishments" – see the variations.

Variation 1: As above, but as soon as the names and the corresponding dice numbers are known to all the game is continued with the cards covered up. If for example a Four is thrown, the man in the top hat is named and the card is turned over. The same is done with all the other cards until all have been turned over. If someone throws the number of a card that has already been turned over, that person goes to the card they think is the right one, names the name and briefly turns it up – for all to see – to check if it is correct, then turns it back over. If they got it wrong, a punishment is of course due.

Variation 2: As above, i.e with visible cards, but when the cards are laid out in a circle an obviously empty space is left. Whoever's turn it is to throw the dice walks or runs to the appropriate card, names it and places it in the empty space, thus creating a new empty space, and the next person does the same. In this way the position of the cards is constantly changed.

Variation 3: A combination of Variations 1 and 2. In other words, the cards are again laid out in a circle with an empty space. One by one the cards are turned over, i.e. the now covered cards constantly change places. The place change is carried out even if the wrong name was named. In this version it is especially important to briefly show everyone the card turned over before moving it, as only in this way will it be possible to more or less have an idea of the current situation.

Variation 4: As in Variation 3, but additional cards are included (they can be the original size). All extra cards – except the nonsense syllable cards – are shuffled and laid face down in the centre of the circle. Anyone who cannot immediately name the card whose number they have thrown draws a card from the deck in the middle and thus receives their task for the "punishment". This task varies, depending on the type of card. The tasks – previously agreed on by the group – are e.g.:

Number card – (here a gymnastic or skipping rope is also needed) add all four numbers and skip as many times as the sum of the numbers on the card!
Letter card – choose one of the eight letters and use this as the first letter of a way of moving, e.g. S for sneak, and move round the circle in this way.
Word card – choose one of the words on the card and mime it until the other players have guessed what it is.
Picture card – mime one of the pictures until the other players have guessed what it is.
Symbol card – (here four gymnastic ropes are needed additionally) choose one of the two graphic symbols and use the ropes to create the form in the centre of the circle.

Variation 5: The whole group, regardless of how big, initially agrees on the names of the six face cards – as in the original version. These are then memorised together with the appropriate dice number. The trainer then disperses the face cards around the room. Now the group runs or walks freely around the room, if desired to music. When the music stops or the trainer gives the signal, everyone stands still and listens to the announcement. Either one of the six names is called out or a number between one and six. As quickly as possible, everyone goes to the appropriate card.

Material: A large foam dice, Nousknacker 2 playing cards; gymnastic ropes for some variations.

Alternating Hideaways

Task: The formation of small groups and the laying out of the six enlarged face cards in a circle as in the original version of "Who's who?" (see page 116) provide the basis here. Additionally, all the other Nousknacker 2 playing cards in their original size are used. They are shuffled well, then one by one a card from the top of the deck of original cards is laid next to each of the face cards in such a way as to be visible to all.

 The rest of the cards are placed in a pile in the centre of the circle. The players now run or walk freely around the room. Each person approaches a face card, spends about ten seconds memorising it in combination with the playing card next to it, moves away and runs briefly about the room before repeating the process with the next card and so on until all six face cards have been memorised. The six playing cards are then pushed under the face cards and are thus no longer visible.

Now the group stands in a circle around the face cards and takes turns at throwing the dice. Whoever throws e.g. a four must remember which card is under the man with the top hat. Is it one with numbers or pictures or perhaps nonsense syllables ... or is it words? In any case, quick decisions are required, for the group counts down in chorus - 5, 4, 3 ... If the dice thrower gets the right answer, she or he can keep the card. If when ... 0 is reached there has been no answer or a wrong answer, the punishment is due without mercy. The face card is lifted. The type of card underneath decides what must be done:

Number card – (here a gymnastic or skipping rope is also needed) add all four numbers and skip as many times as the sum of the numbers on the card!

Letter card – choose one of the eight letters and use this as the first letter of a way of moving, e.g. S for sneak, and move round the circle in this way.
Word card – choose one of the words on the card and mime it until the other players have guessed what it is.
Picture card – mime one of the pictures until the other players have guessed what it is.
Symbol card – (here four gymnastic ropes are needed additionally) choose one of the two graphic symbols and use the ropes to create the form in the centre of the circle.

When the punishment has been carried out, the card is put in the middle of the circle. The only exception: the nonsense syllable card. The player now has another chance to win the card. He or she must study the card for ten seconds and then correctly name and spell all four syllables.

Before the dice is passed on, the player draws a new card from the pile in the middle and quickly goes around the inside of the circle holding the card for all to see. Only then does she or he put the card under the now "vacant" face card. Who has gathered the most cards by the end of the game?

Variation: As above, but when the person whose turn it is cannot win the card, others can have a try. The first to get at least one character right – a number, letter, picture ... – gets to keep the card. Of course it has to be named before the punishment is carried out!

Material: A large foam dice, Nousknacker 2 playing cards; four gymnastic ropes for some variations.

Note: The six face cards from Nousknacker 2 should be available in enlarged form. Alternatively six large faces can be cut out of magazines, stuck on cardboard and have dice numbers from one to six put on them. The other playing cards - as far as they are needed – can be used in the original size.

In all forms of moving Nousknacker the different types of movement can and should be varied. Whenever walking or running is called for, the trainer should determine whether the direction should be forwards, backwards or sideways. The length of steps and the pace are other ways of varying the movement. Additional difficulties can be created with obstacles or by balancing materials.

10 Brain Training in Clubs

10.1 Another New Sports Idea?

Is the club really the right place for brain training? Shouldn't it be offered by completely different organisations? Should the club now do that as well? These and other questions are sure to be asked by many when they hear the topic. Therefore let it be made quite clear again: Brain training is not a new offer for the club. As a rule it is not offered in special sessions set up extra, but is integrated in existing programmes. Many of the exercises have already been done for quite some time, but with a different purpose, only being considered from the point of view of movement. This applies to many gymnastic and sports programmes.

Gymnastics and sport mainly pick up the topic of brain training because one of their important tasks is to publicly demonstrate the positive effects of gymnastics and sport, i.e. of club activities. In order for this to take place, many trainers have to first be made aware that their work covers more than purely physical aspects.

Clubs can thus continue their programmes as in the past, perhaps supplementing them if they wish. Above all though they should intensively make use of their opportunity to develop a consciousness of the significance of brain training. When trainers inform themselves about brain training, it can result in them making changes to the content of their lessons, using certain exercises more consciously and possibly changing the order of the exercises in order to make better use of the thinking capacity of their members.

An important aspect of the club is its function as a focal point, as a meeting and communication centre. The trainer is a person people have confidence in and seek advice from on questions and problems that go beyond matters of sport. It is often expected of such persons in a consulting role that they have information available on general topics regarding health and fitness.

Memory training, brain jogging, brain performance training – these are subjects being discussed more and more often, especially amongst older people who are often afraid of decreasing mental performance. Anyone training a group of adults cannot be an expert in all these fields but should at least have heard of them and have an idea of what they involve. Also it should be known that training the short term memory has priority for people who are not so young anymore.

Some clubs – so one finds already – would like to do more in the field of brain training. Such activities can easily be integrated in the programmes of many clubs in the areas of health and fitness, if sufficient capacity is available. The links between exercise and thinking are clearly evident. For many clubs it is therefore the obvious thing to do, to profit from the opportunities these links offer. Frequently people want to find things that belong together - such as exercise and thinking - in the same place - in their club. It is particularly important for older people, who are no longer as mobile as they once were, to find an attractive programme being offered by a club nearby which has their confidence. Experiencing new and unknown things – like brain jogging/brain performance training – in familiar surroundings together with a group already familiar from gymnastics training can help remove initial hesitation of sceptics. Some clubs have added introductory courses in brain jogging/brain performance training to their usual programme and have found strong interest among their members. It is perfectly all right for younger and older people to train their mental fitness together. It is, however, important that such courses are run by someone specially trained to do so. After all, no club would like it if untrained personnel suddenly began running courses in gymnastics and sport. Section 10.3 "Prerequisites and qualification" contains more about the necessary qualifications.

10.2 Forms of Organisation and Presentation for Brain Jogging/Brain Performance Training/Mental Activation Training

The club is really the ideal place for special programmes like brain jogging in addition to its sporting activities. It is ideal because it has the opportunity – unlike many other organisations – to give its members not only an introduction to the techniques but above all to motivate them to permanently practise these. Most courses offered in other locations usually involve eight training units as an introduction. After that, each participant is left on their own. But even very intensive brain training is of little use if it is not done regularly. After all, physically it is just as little use to achieve the standards necessary for an award once a year and then spend the rest of the year inactively. Regular practice is decisive – both for body and mind.

The club with its group and its community offers a feeling of belonging and creates motivation. It removes initial fears when starting and helps develop enjoyment when people carry on. It is important to create a consciousness amongst all members that we ourselves are very much responsible not only for a healthy body but also for a healthy mind.

If a club wishes to make use of its ideal prerequisites and in addition to other organisations to include brain jogging or brain performance training/ mental activation training in its programme, it should be clear right from the start that a specially trained person is necessary. The club should therefore take advantage of possibilities arising through useful cooperations. The following concrete possibilities are available to clubs:

* Carry out a one-off information event (c. 90 minutes) run by a trained expert* as an initial introduction to the subject for members and potential members as a special event.

* Carry out a course on brain jogging/ brain performance training/ mental activation training run by a trained expert* under the auspices of the club. A course generally involves eight afternoon or evening sessions of 90 minutes duration each.

* Joint attendance with the club of a course offered by another organisation.

* After doing the course together: Ten minutes brain performance training together in connection with the usual sport session, i.e. before or after it.

* Mutual motivation and "success tracking" by doing and comparing brain jogging "homework" between club sessions.

* Development of cooperation between club trainers and brain training experts or cooperation between organisations involved in the two aspects.

- Send interested club members – not necessarily just trainers! – to training courses in the field of brain training.

(necessary qualification: see section "Prerequisites and qualification"

10.3 Prerequisites and Qualification

The ideal general prerequisites for brain jogging/ brain performance training/ mental activation training in clubs have been extensively described. Here now are the concrete requirements with regard to location and personnel.

For special courses in brain jogging/ brain performance training/ mental activation training a group room with tables and chairs is needed, not a hall. The group should be comprised of about twelve people. The space required corresponds to this. It is ideal but not absolutely necessary to have a small open space next to the tables and chairs for movement games etc. Classrooms in schools are often good for this. Here though, one should make sure there are tables and chairs for adults as sitting and working at children's furniture is anything but good for one's health!

For training short term memory – as already extensively demonstrated – the method of brain performance training/ mental activation training is especially suitable. In Germany two training organisations are nationally responsible for training experts in this method:

1. WissIOMed-Ausbildungsstätte Memory-Klinik Nordrach Klausenbach
2. Gesellschaft für Gehirntraining (GfG) with its Trainer College.

Both organisations have an up to date database of trained experts who can carry out courses in brain performance training/ mental activation training. On request they can provide addresses of appropriate persons close to interested clubs.

At both organisations the training course for instructors to run courses for healthy people corresponds in type and comprehensiveness approximately to the training to run sports sessions, i.e. it is not necessary to hold a special occupational qualification. On the other hand, for a course to carry out brain function training with people who are ill, an occupational qualification is required.

The Memory-Klinik Nordrach Klausenbach (Germany) with the WisslOMed trains its students as
• Assistant for brain performance training for healthy persons FAH®
• Assistant for brain performance training for healthy persons FAH® specialised in movement (Cooperation: DTB-Akademie + Memory-Klinik Nordrach Klausenbach with the WisslOMed; acceptance only with valid DSB licence or professional sports qualification)
• Expert for brain function training for ill persons FKH® (Acceptance only with appropriate professional qualification).

The course of the "Gesellschaft für Gehirntraining (GfG)" with its trainer college finishes with brain trainer licences
    • Licence C for carrying out courses for healthy persons and
    • Licence B for carrying out individual therapy for ill persons.

There are a number of other organisations involved in training trainers. Most of them teach the memory training method of Dr. med Franziska Stengel which has already been described. Information is available from the "Bundesverband Gedächtnistraining".

All addresses : see chapter "Addresses", page 139.

11 Appendix

Crossing Out Numbers

Cross out the numbers from 1 - 22 in ascending order, i.e. first 1, then 2, then 3 etc. in the following number pattern!

		10	4
	7		
22	11	20	16
14	1	21	6
8	19		18
		2	
17	15	9	12
	13		
3		5	

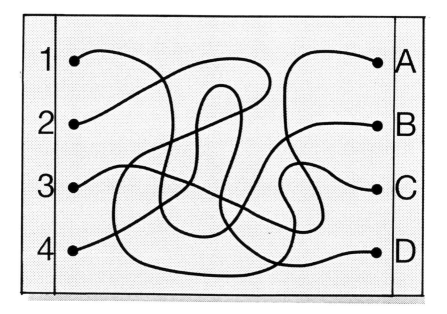

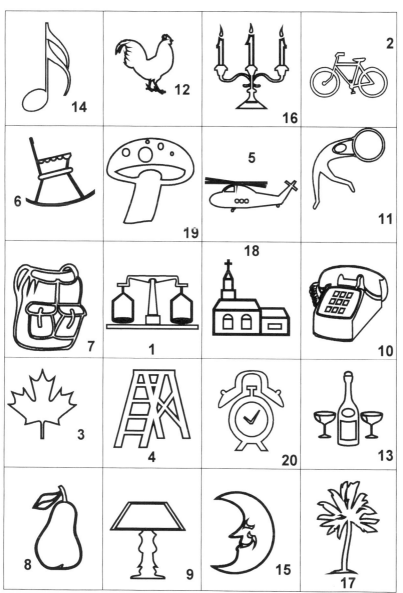

(created by Bettina M. Jasper with Cliparts from Corel Draw, Corel Corporation, Canada)

The Brain Fitness Circuit - Thinking and Movement at 1 + 10 Stations
Game List

Name:

Station 1: Picture Board
1. Walking/Fast walking/Running on the spot
2. Memorise 20 pictures, where appropriate with numbers

Station 2: Peggy Sue
1. Move forwards pegged together as a pair
2. Find words in the alphabet square

Station 3: Buttonhole
1. Do up as many buttons as possible
2. Cross out number patterns

Station 4: Bucket Run
1. Run to look at seven letters hidden under buckets
2. First write the letters here, then sort them

Station 5: Parts of a Whole
1. Screw together ballpoint pens "blindly"
2. Put together puzzle

Station 6: Ball Test
1. Throw ball at wall and catch it
2. Read text with spelling mistakes

Station 7: Feeling Box
1. Feel objects and write down here what they are
   _____

2. Look intensely at poster "Picture Board" again intensely and add up the numbers in the 20 spaces. Result:
   _____

Station 8: Noticeboard
1. Move forwards with a sheet of newspaper against one's chest without it falling
2. Cross out all capital and small "A"s and "a"s

Station 9: Buttoneyes
1. Sort buttons into pairs and threes
2. Study the "Chessboard" pattern for c. 10 seconds then copy it here:

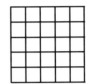

Station 10: Balancing Act
1. Balance along a bench or a line, changing direction as often as possible without leaving the object
2. Find terms about subject X with the right number of syllables and write them here:

1 syllable	
2 syllables	
3 syllables	
4 syllables	
5 syllables	

Station 11: Rope Walking
1. Rope walking and counting the strokes
2. Memorise as many as possible of the 20 pictures and put them in the right position here, if possible with the appropriate number:

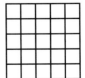

(created by Bettina M. Jasper with Cliparts from Corel Draw, Corel Corporation, Canada)

Alphabet Square

The following words are hidden horizontally, vertically and diagonally in the alphabet square:
gymnastics, symbol, brain, sign, training, mind, movement, word, club, thoughts, golf, sense, fitness, number, jogging, picture.

Find the words and circle them!

D	N	S	T	H	G	U	O	H	T	U	X	T
U	Z	G	S	S	R	C	W	O	R	D	S	E
F	Y	S	I	K	A	S	T	B	A	V	B	S
S	S	C	N	S	S	E	N	T	I	F	C	E
M	L	I	M	Y	N	L	D	Y	N	A	L	N
O	R	T	H	M	I	B	R	A	I	N	U	S
V	N	S	I	B	I	P	Z	Y	N	F	B	E
E	E	A	V	O	G	N	I	U	G	E	N	K
M	F	N	E	L	I	R	D	C	U	L	E	W
E	U	M	R	H	J	P	B	O	T	F	N	A
N	A	Y	E	D	S	R	E	B	M	U	N	B
T	E	G	N	I	G	G	o	J	M	I	R	T
R	U	V	N	T	S	I	E	G	R	W	I	E

Crossing Out Number Patterns

Example: 96⁄2
            1⁄2⁄3
            ⁄2⁄3⁄7
            ⁄3⁄49
            ⁄438

Column 1	Column 2	Column 3	Column 4
985	183	398	329
498	985	498	293
387	091	871	209
853	109	583	409
490	291	928	395
402	964	307	555
218	349	295	517
258	472	390	605
309	309	406	209
877	485	086	398
908	984	290	294
219	298	234	460
098	298	583	298
971	089	409	371
290	857	089	743
593	395	498	456
875	345	222	345
358	847	624	239
583	984	205	490
209	456	345	989
108	349	984	345
394	348	457	309
309	853	982	724
093	982	345	982
938	973	728	803
198	298	340	348
309	345	540	308
892	793	340	809
837	398	490	345
530	456	793	364
987	345	862	503

Scrambled Letters: "Sports"

Re-sort the letters below. In the right order, each line is a different sport. Write the solutions next to the mixed letters.

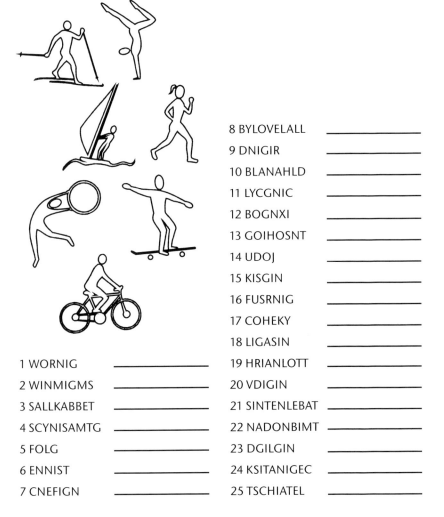

8 BYLOVELALL   _____

9 DNIGIR   _____

10 BLANAHLD   _____

11 LYCGNIC   _____

12 BOGNXI   _____

13 GOIHOSNT   _____

14 UDOJ   _____

15 KISGIN   _____

16 FUSRNIG   _____

17 COHEKY   _____

18 LIGASIN   _____

1 WORNIG   _____ 19 HRIANLOTT   _____

2 WINMIGMS   _____ 20 VDIGIN   _____

3 SALLKABBET   _____ 21 SINTENLEBAT   _____

4 SCYNISAMTG   _____ 22 NADONBIMT   _____

5 FOLG   _____ 23 DGILGIN   _____

6 ENNIST   _____ 24 KSITANIGEC   _____

7 CNEFIGN   _____ 25 TSCHIATEL   _____

"Spelling Mistakes"

In the following text by Ernest Hemingway there are many spelling mistakes. Try to read it anyway! Replace each symbol with a letter.

"N❶ck dr➤p◀ed c♣ref♥lly d♠wn the emb♫nk♥ent ♠nd cut i❺to the w♦ods t❹ co♫e up t➡ the f♦re thr♠ugh th♦ tre♣s. It w♥s a b⑧ech♠o⑦d f♫rest ❾nd the f♣llcn beec♫nut b♠rrs w♥re ♦nder his sh♣es as he w♣lked betw♦en the tre❸s. The f♦re w♣s br♦ght n♣w, j♥st at the ♫dge of the tre♦s. Th◀re w⑧s a m♣n sitt♠ng by it. N♥ck w◀ited b♫hind th♥ trees and w♦tched. The m♠n looked t♣ be al♫ne. H❸ w♦s si♠ting th♣re w◀th his h♦ad in his h♫nds lo⑧king ♥t the f♦re. N♦ck st⑧pped out ♥nd w◀lked ♦nto the fir♣light. The m♫n s♠t th⑧re lo♦king ♦nto th♣ f❸re. Wh♦n Nick stop♥ed q⑧ite cl♣se to h♦m he d♥d n♫t m❸ve."

From: Ernest Hemingway, The Battler

"Chessboard" Pattern

Right Number of Syllables

Here one has to look for the right numbers of syllables. For each subject a term must be found with one syllable, one with two, three ... up to five syllables. Write any suitable terms with the appropriate number of syllables on the lines – the subject is written above them in each case.

Example: **Bicycle**
1 syllable   2 syllables   3 syllables   4 syllables   5 syllables
Tube   sad-dle   dy-na-mo   bi-cy-cle-stand   ra-cing-bi-cy-cle

Rainy weather

_____   _____   _____   _____   _____

Church

_____   _____   _____   _____   _____

Jeweller

_____   _____   _____   _____   _____

Football

_____   _____   _____   _____   _____

Farm

_____   _____   _____   _____   _____

Laundry

_____   _____   _____   _____   _____

Politics

_____   _____   _____   _____   _____

Toys

_____   _____   _____   _____   _____

Insects

_____   _____   _____   _____   _____

Television

_____   _____   _____   _____   _____

12 Bibliography and Addresses

Bibliography

Baumann, Hartmut/Leye, Monika (Hrsg.): Das SIMA-Projekt: Psycho-motorisches Training. Hofgrefe Verlag, Kempten 1995, ISBN 3-8017-0813-6.

Fischer, Bernd/Lehrl, Siegfried/Lehrl, Maria/Mosmann, Hannjette: GeJo Card, 50 Spielkarten (Zahlen) mit Anleitung und Spielblock. Vless Verlag, Ebersberg, ISBN 3-88562-046-4.

Fischer, Bernd/Lehrl, Siegfried: Selber denken macht fit. Vless Verlag, Ebersberg, 1990, 2. Aufl., ISBN 3-88562-039-1.

Fischer, Bernd/Dickreiter, Bernhard/Mosmann, Hannjette: Fit ab Fünfzig! Vitalitätskonzept. Haslach 1996, ISBN 3-9804146-5-5.

Fischer, Bernd/Dickreiter, Bernhard: Geistige Fitness Hirt Institut, Zürich, 1994.

Jasper, Bettina M.: Fit im Kopf. Gehirn-Jogging als mentales Aktivierungstraining. In: Deutscher Turner-Bund; Gesundheitssport für Ältere, Frankfurt 1993, ISBN 3-929461-20-x.

Jasper, Bettina M.: Bewegung fördern. Reihe: Aktives Alter – Gekonnt betreuen und aktivieren. Vincentz Verlag, Hannover, 1993, ISBN 3-87870-406-2.

Jasper, Bettina M.: Spiel und Gespräch. Reihe: Aktives Alter – Gekonnt betreuen und aktivieren. Vincentz Verlag, Hannover, 1995, ISBN 3-87870-025-3.

Lehrl, Siegfried: GeJo Letra, 55 Spielkarten (Buchstaben) mit Anleitung und Spielblock. Vless Verlag, Ebersberg, ISBN 3-88562-047-2.

Lehrl, Siegfried/Fischer, Bernd/Lehrl, Maria; Reihe Gehirntraining: GeJo-Leitfaden. Ein Überblick über Gehirn-Jogging – Grundlagen und Anwendungen. Vless Verlag, Ebersberg, 1990, ISBN 3-88562-037-5.

Lehrl, Siegfried/Fischer, Bernd/Koch, Gerhard/Loddenkemper, Hermann; Gehirn-Jogging. Geist und Gedächtnis erfolgreich trainieren. Mediteg Verlag, Wehrheim, 1992, 6. Aufl., ISBN 3-924373-10-8.

Mosmann, Hannjette/Fischer, Bernd/Dickreiter, Bernhard: Nousknacker 1, Gehirn-Jogging-Kartenspiel, 64 Spielkarten mit Begleitheft. Nordrach 1995.

Mosmann, Hannjette/Fischer, Bernd/Dickreiter, Bernhard: Nousknacker 2, Gehirn-Jogging-Kartenspiel, 64 Spielkarten und 1 Würfel mit Begleitheft. Nordrach 1995.

Oswald, Wolf D./Rödel, Gisela: Das SIMA-Projekt: Gedächtnistraining. Hofgrefe Verlag, Kempten 1995, ISBN 3-8017-0818-7.
Stengel, Franziska; Gedächtnis spielend trainieren. 33 Spielarten mit 333 Spielen. Memo Verlag Hedwig Ladner, Stuttgart 1993, 7. Aufl., ISBN 3-929317-84-2.

Various exercise books and material for training of brain fitness/mental activity are available at

Denk-Werkstatt®, Sasbachwalden
Mediteg Verlag, Wehrheim
Vless-Verlag, Ebersberg
WissIOMed GmbH, Nordrach

Adresses
Deutscher Turner-Bund (DTB)
Otto-Fleck-Schneise 8
60528 Frankfurt am Main
Tel.   069/67 80 1-0
Fax   069/67 80 1-179

DTB-Akademie
Otto-Fleck-Schneise 8
60528 Frankfurt am Main
Tel.   069/67 80 1-0
Fax   069/67 80 1-179

Memory Liga e.V.
Präsident: Prof. Dr. Bernd Fischer
c/o Memory-Klinik Klausenbach
Kolonie 5
77787 Nordrach
Tel.   07838/82-0
Fax   07838/707

WissIOMed GmbH
Postfach 7
77785 Nordrach
Tel.   07838/658
Fax   07838/707

Gesellschaft für Gehirntraining (GfG)
Präsident: Dr. Siegfried Lehrl
Postfach 1460
85555 Ebersberg
Tel.   08092/2 41 24
Fax   08092/2 03 67

GfG Trainer-Kolleg für Mentale Aktivierung GmbH
Marienplatz 6
85560 Ebersberg
Tel.   08092/2 04 38
Fax   08092/2 03 67

Bundesverband Gedächtnistraining nach Dr. med. Franziska Stengel e.V.
Zum Appelhof 1
51570 Windeck-Herchen
Tel.   02243/3443
Fax   02243/3443

Denk-Werkstatt
Rebblick 5
77887 Sasbachwalden
Tel.   07841/2 81 09
Fax   07841/2 81 09

Mediteg Verlag
Limesstr. 5
61273 Wehrheim
Tel.   06081/5171 + 5 60 17
Fax   06081/5 60 17

Vincentz Verlag
Postfach 6247
30062 Hannover
Tel.   0511/9910-033
Fax   0511/9910-039

Vless Verlag
Marienplatz 4
85560 Ebersberg
Tel.   08092/2 10 53
Fax   08092/2 03 67

Journal "New Studies in Athletics"
Coaching Tips for Children's Soccer
Soccer Training Programmes
Training Exercises for Competitive Tennis
Advanced Techniques for Competitive Tennis
Running to the Top
Distance Training for Young Athletes
Modern Sports Karate
Scientific Coaching for Olympic Taekwondo
Handbook for Beach Volleyball
Handbook of Competitive Cycling
The Complete Guide to Duathlon Training
Triathlon Training
Allround Fitness – The Beginner's Guide
Teaching Children's Gymnastics – Spotting and Securing
Train Your Brain – Mental and Physical Fitness
Straight Golf – The Basics of Good Golf
Contact Improvisation – Moving, Dancing, Interaction
Jazz Dance Training
Big Foot – A Complete Guide
Integration through Games and Sports
Recreational Games and Tournaments
Sport Sciences in Europe 1993 – Current and Future Perspectives
Physical Education and Sport – Changes and Challenges
Racism and Xenophobia in European Football
The CSRC-Edition Volumes 1-6
Physical Activity for Life: East and West, South and North
Physical Education: A Reader
Cultural Diversity and Congruence in Physical Education and Sport

MEYER & MEYER SPORT

Von-Coels-Str. 390 · D-52080 Aachen · Tel. 0241/9 58 10-0 · Fax 0241/9 58 10-10
e-mail: verlag@meyer-meyer-sports.com • http://www.meyer-meyer-sports.com